Y0-CDC-694

Second Edition, September, 2001

Good Health - Do It Yourself! Copyright 2001 by Matthias Rath, M.D.
All rights reserved. Published by MR Publishing, Inc., Santa Clara, CA 95054
No part of this book may be used or reproduced in any manner whatsoever without
written permission except in the case of brief quotations embodied in critical articles
or reviews. For information: editor@drrath.com

This book is not intended to substitute for the medical advice of a physician.
The reader should regularly consult a physician in matters relating to his or her health and
particularly in respect to any symptoms that may require diagnosis or medical attention.
The authors and the publisher disclaim responsibility for any adverse effects resulting
directly or indirectly from the information contained in this book.

RSA10021

ISBN 0-9638768-7-2

Good Health - Do It Yourself!

Matthias Rath, M.D.

Contents

Foreword

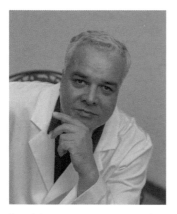

This book is dedicated to the many thousands of consultants who have passed on the vital information about Cellular Health in Germany among other countries. It is our common goal to build up a new health system, one that finally serves the interests of the people.

This book constitutes the final strike against a falsely conceived health system. It proves that endemic diseases, under the influence of the pharmaceutical industry, have artificially been kept alive for a hundred years as global markets for mostly ineffective and dangerous pharmaceutical treatments.

This book proves that the most significant "common diseases" of today are not diseases at all but the inevitable consequence of years of deficiency in vitamins and other natural substances whose function is essential to the metabolism of millions of body cells.

This book lays the foundation for insuring that heart attacks, strokes, high blood pressure, cardiac insufficiency, diabetic complications, and other diseases, will soon become a thing of the past.

This book is the signpost for any courageous politician to stand up for fundamental reform of the healthcare system. Above all, those untenable laws that form an obstacle to the spread of this vital information must be eliminated.

This book is also the answer for doctors and other members of the healthcare professions who have recognized the dead end streets of conventional medicine and are opening up new routes. Cellular Health is the basis for the health care of the future.

Above all, this book is the answer for hundreds of millions of patients all over the world who for decades have been at the mercy of the pharmaceutical industry and the blind alleys of outmoded medicine. Here is the answer to their health problems.

We invite you to join us in building a new healthcare system by broadcasting the information in this book wherever you go. Pass the book on to your friends, acquaintances, colleagues, and neighbors. Take it to your club, church, or other groups. Give it as a birthday present – instead of flowers. Give it to your doctor, or have it displayed in their offices.

You will be helping other people and saving lives.
This book was written by patients and those afflicted. It is to them that we owe our thanks. This book is only the beginning; documentation of the success of Cellular Health continues and will one day fill whole shelves. Send us your report for the next edition of this book. You will be helping many people by doing this.

My thanks go to Angelika Zuta-Sadovic, Marian Peters, and Christina Rauch for collating and processing the texts, and in particular to Dirk Brandt for coordinating the compilation of the documentation.

Matthias Rath M.D.

INTRODUCTION
Cellular Health – a breakthrough in the natural prevention and causal therapy of common diseases

Matthias Rath, M.D. is considered the founder of Cellular Health, the new understanding that most common diseases are based on a deficient vitamin supply to millions of body cells. This new concept of health and disease is the basis for the remarkable success stories documented in this book. The scientific principles of Cellular Health are summarized below.

The cells in our body perform a multitude of functions: glandular cells produce hormones, white blood corpuscles manufacture antibodies, and heart muscle cells produce electrical energy for the heart to beat. The specific task of each cell is determined by the genetic code in the cell nucleus comparable to a metabolism software program. Although these tasks may be very different, each cell uses the same bioenergy sources (biological catalysts) for a multitude of vital biochemical reactions within the cell. Many of these biological catalysts cannot be produced by the body itself. They must be taken externally as supplements.

Vitamins, minerals, trace elements, and certain amino acids are of particular importance here. The most important of these essential biological catalysts are summarized in Dr. Rath's research. Without the regular and optimal supply of these bioenergy sources, functional deficiency of the cells, organ malfunction, and subsequently disease are the result.

The constituents of a sound vitamin program catalyze thousands of biochemical reactions in each cell

The most important biological catalysts

- Vitamin C
- Vitamin B-1
- Vitamin B-2
- Vitamin B-3
- Vitamin B-4
- Vitamin B-5
- Vitamin B-6
- Vitamin B-12
- Carnitine*
- Coenzyme Q-10
- Minerals
- Trace elements

Single cell

Energy center (mitochondrion)

Cell "software" center (nucleus)

Cell production center (endoplasmatic reticulum)

The metabolism software program in each cell is determined precisely by the genetic information in the cell nucleus.

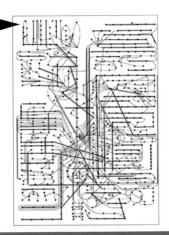

The constituents of the vitamin program are used as biological catalysts and bioenergy sources in each cell. They are indispensable for the optimal functioning of millions of cells.

Cellular Health Helps Keep Heart and Circulatory Disease in Check

Cellular Health forms the scientific basis for winning the battle against death from heart disease. The correlations are easy enough to understand. The heart and circulatory system are the mechanically most active organ systems in our body. As a result of the constant pumping action to maintain blood circulation, the cells of the circulatory system have a particularly high turnover in cell energy and a particularly high consumption of vitamins and other biological catalysts.

First of all, the most important types of cells making up the heart and circulatory system include:

• **The cells of the blood vessel walls:** The endothelial cells form the barrier between the bloodstream and blood vessel wall. These cells contribute to a variety of metabolic functions, such as optimal viscosity. The smooth muscle cells produce collagen and are responsible for optimal stability and elasticity of the blood vessel walls.

• **The cells of the heart muscle:** The principal task of the heart muscle cells is to ensure the pumping function of the heart. Furthermore, some of the muscle cells are specialized to produce and conduct electrical stimuli for the heartbeat.

• **The blood cells:** Millions of blood corpuscles circulating in our blood are nothing more than cells. They are responsible for transporting oxygen, for resistance to diseases and the elimination of waste, for the healing of wounds, and other functions.

The cardiovascular system is composed of millions of cells

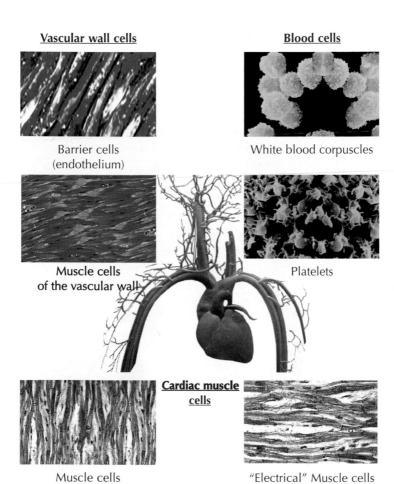

Vascular wall cells

Barrier cells
(endothelium)

Muscle cells
of the vascular wall

Blood cells

White blood corpuscles

Platelets

Cardiac muscle cells

Muscle cells
for pumping action

"Electrical" Muscle cells
for heartbeat

11

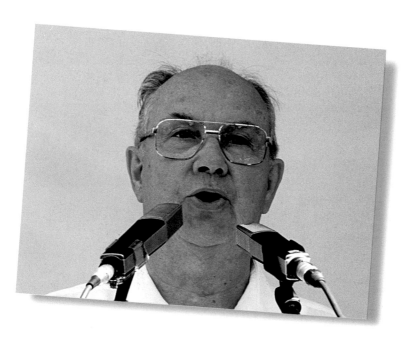

**One of many who testified to the benefits
of vitamin therapy**

1

- **Heart Attack**
- **Stroke**
- **Hardening of the Arteries**
- **Circulatory Problems**

**Cellular Health
for Natural Prevention
and Health Maintenance**

The Facts About Coronary Heart Disease

- **Every year, every other death in the industrialized world** is due to atherosclerotic deposits in the coronary arteries (leading to heart attack) or in the arteries supplying blood to the brain (leading to stroke). The epidemic spread of these cardiovascular diseases is largely due to the fact that until now the true nature of atherosclerosis and coronary heart disease has not been understood.

- **Conventional medicine** is largely confined to treating the symptoms of this disease. Calcium antagonists, beta-blockers, nitrates, and other drugs are prescribed to alleviate angina pain. Surgical procedures (angioplasty, bypass surgery) are applied to improve blood flow mechanically. Hardly any conventional medicine targets the underlying problem: the instability of the vascular wall which triggers the development of atherosclerotic deposits.

- **Cellular Health** provides a breakthrough in our understanding of these causes and leads to effective prevention and treatment of coronary heart disease. The primary cause of coronary heart disease and other forms of atherosclerotic disease is a chronic deficiency of vitamins and other essential nutrients in millions of vascular wall cells. This leads to instability of the vascular walls, to lesions and cracks, to atherosclerotic deposits, and eventually to heart attacks or strokes. Since the primary cause of cardiovascular disease is a deficiency of essential nutrients in the vascular wall, a daily optimum intake of these essential nutrients is the primary measure to prevent atherosclerosis and to help repair vascular wall damage.

Heart attack, stroke, atherosclerosis

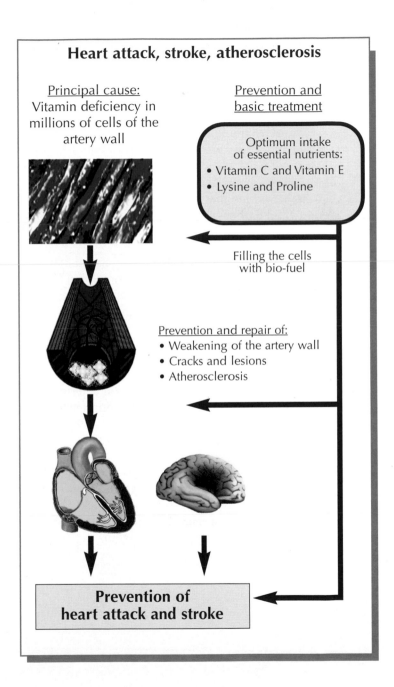

Principal cause:
Vitamin deficiency in millions of cells of the artery wall

Prevention and basic treatment

Optimum intake of essential nutrients:
- Vitamin C and Vitamin E
- Lysine and Proline

Filling the cells with bio-fuel

Prevention and repair of:
- Weakening of the artery wall
- Cracks and lesions
- Atherosclerosis

Prevention of heart attack and stroke

Dear Dr. Rath,

This time last year I had just had an operation after a stroke. I only survived this stroke without further damage because the operation was carried out quickly and by an experienced angioplasty surgeon. Calcified blockages were removed from both carotid arteries. But what about the calcium in the smaller arteries, in my brain and feet and heart? The senior consultant told me that another operation was not possible and further blocking of the arteries must be prevented.

When I left hospital my son recommended that I accompany him to a lecture to hear something about correct diet and vitamins. We then began taking vitamins and minerals after studying your books.

This produced the following verifiable results to the astonishment of all the doctors treating me:

• **No new calcification of the carotid arteries was found** but, on the contrary, **decalcification** ensued. These were the findings in May this year at the clinic where I had the operation in July last year.

• I have been diabetic since 1986 and already had **circulatory problems in my legs and feet**. These have **almost disappeared**. No more cold feet. The extremely high **blood sugar level** has considerably been reduced; the level is **normal again**.

• My **eyes** have improved; the **internal pressure is normal again.**

• Heart complaints, particularly at night, have gone, and I can sleep well. Also, my previously diagnosed **arrhythmia has gone**. My short-term memory has improved. I can solve normal crossword puzzles, one after the other.

• There has also been a considerable improvement for my wife who has suffered from migraine and painful joints for years. Also her **blood pressure is normal again.**

All in all we have a new lease on life, can deal with our age with much more optimism, and are less afraid about the future. For us, a new life has begun. I am 65 years old and feel like 50 again!

Yours sincerely,

W.B.

Dear Dr. Rath,

I am 61 years old and have been suffering from **angina pectoris** for four years. I have obviously inherited the susceptibility from my father. I was plagued and restricted by sudden **shortage of breath** at the slightest exertion. In January last year I had a **bypass operation**.

I heard of your work and I began taking vitamins and nutritional supplements on 14th of June last year. After twelve weeks I had no pains any more, not even with increased exertion. **I no longer feel pressure on the heart or breathlessness** which I still had after the operation! My **blood pressure** has returned to **normal** since December last year, the operation scars have healed well, today there are no pains from the scars at all.

After the last electron radiation tomography at the University Clinic Erlangen-Nürnberg the doctors there diagnosed my condition as follows: "Given the subjective absence of symptoms and good resilience, we can see **no indication of any progression of the coronary heart disease which was present.**" The atherosclerosis which caused me so much trouble has therefore actually been halted.

I feel absolutely fit. The acid test was when I was able to lift 40-kg sacks up a ladder onto a 10-m high scaffolding.

I am thankful I heard about nutritional therapy. It has saved my life **and all without any side effects!** I don't need medicines any more now!

Yours sincerely,

Werner Wolf

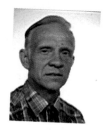

Dear Dr. Rath,

In the fall of 1995 my uncle's health deteriorated so much (he is 94 years old) that it became necessary to dilate various **constrictions in his coronary arteries**. He has had heart problems since he was a child. By the end of 1994 there were periods of **extremely high blood pressure** that was supposed to be cured by medicines. All in vain!

The first dilatation of the constriction was successful and my uncle was able to lead a relatively pleasant life again. Sadly, this was only for barely three months. Then the attacks were worse than before. A particularly critical point (bend) had again become constricted and attempts to dilate this spot failed.

In the spring of 1996 my uncle was referred to Bad Oeynhausen, where it was possible to open up this spot again minimally but only on the second attempt. My uncle was then discharged.

As was to be expected, his health deteriorated month by month. More medicines were added and finally only constant spraying with "Nitro" kept him alive somehow.

Working in the garden or manual activities were out of the question. **Heart attacks and periods of high blood pressure characterized his daily life.** The thought of dying soon haunted him constantly.

This was the condition until March last year when I received your book. After reading it feverishly one evening I decided to supplement my diet with vitamins and minerals. My uncle also supplemented his diet.

To date my uncle has had no need to take these drops! **His condition improved week by week.** He noticed that he could also do physical things again, such as bending without falling over. Several weeks later my uncle got on his bicycle and made an (accompanied) **cycling trip without difficulty.** I could give you many more examples of the positive changes in my uncle.

Yours sincerely,

B.K.

Dear Dr. Rath,

Since learning of Cellular Health, I have been taking a vitamin program since September 1996, I would like to tell you about it today.

My dear wife sadly passed away following heart attacks in 1970 and 1991—in February 1996.
I have been suffering for a long time from **angina pectoris and have had several dilatations** (widening of the blood vessels), the last one about four months after the death of my wife. During my subsequent stay in the hospital, I read a small article in the "Welt am Sonntag" introducing your book. The next day I ordered the book from my bookshop and did not rest until I had finished reading it. My GP, whom I asked for advice, advised me to take the preparation. I ordered it and waited.

Finally on the morning of my departure to the North of Germany, the postman brought me the long-awaited package. I threw it into the waiting car and drove off. I began taking the basic course of treatment at the house of my friends in Husum. **After a week**, when I started my journey home,
I was already a new man; I felt much better and drove all 900 km home without stopping. On the way there I had been forced to make an overnight stay.

From then my health improved again. I spent the following winter in Tenerife.

In the summer of last year I was again sent to hospital. The coronary angiograph only showed a slight deposit in one of the coronary arteries. **No further dilatation was necessary. In spring this year I had the laboratory results checked. The results were all excellent.**

I attribute the fact that I am so well again today to vitamins and minerals and for this I would like to give my heartfelt thanks to you, Dr. Rath, and your team. In the meantime I have told many of my acquaintances about the program and I believe I can say, with success.

I am only sad that I didn't know about you and your research years ago; maybe I would have been able to help my wife.

Again, many thanks,

Yours sincerely,

H.S.

Dear Dr. Rath,

I am 53 years old, and eight years ago I had an **infarction of the anterior wall**. After this I constantly had feelings of anxiety and occasionally **high blood pressure**. On the 1st of March last year I began taking a vitamin regimen after reading one of your books.

After four to five months I felt **considerably more capable. I have stopped taking all medicines such as beta-blockers and ASS 100.**

Until now, no doctor to this date has been able to explain why I had a heart attack. I did not have any of the risk factors, as I am a nonsmoker and I am not overweight.

Yours faithfully,

V.S.

Dear Dr. Rath,

I am 47 years old and for two years have been suffering from **angina pectoris**. I was plagued by **sweating, shortage of breath, nausea, and pains in the thorax** and in my left arm.

Two months ago I began supplementing my diet with vitamins and minerals following the principles of Cellular Health. After only three weeks I only felt a slight pressure in the chest, but **no more shortage of breath, and nausea and outbreaks of sweat have totally disappeared.**

I would like to thank you, Dr. Rath, and I will tell other people about Cellular Health.

Yours sincerely,

Ursula Rösner

Dear Dr. Rath,

About two years ago I suffered **cardiac infarction** as a result of the passing away of my dear wife after a long period of care.

After that I had constant problems with **angina pectoris, a burning feeling with pressure, and a feeling of tightness in the chest**. By taking vitamins, minerals, trace elements, and coenzyme Q10, which were recommended to me, I was able to keep the problems somewhat in check but could not stop them.

Of course I had completely changed my diet too, but the angina pectoris symptoms, and above all the feelings of anxiety that prevented me from sleeping at night made taking medicine for sleep inevitable.

I am 78 years old and want to get rid of these complaints. As this was not possible through medicine and the fact that the attending **doctor advised balloon catheter treatment**, I decided to find a natural treatment to avoid surgery.

An acquaintance explained Cellular Health to me. I also read your book and saw it as a last chance for me to avoid a coronary angioplasty operation.

2

At the beginning of May this year I began taking vitamins and minerals, starting slowly at first. I continued to consult my doctor.

Already after only two weeks I noticed a distinct improvement. The burning sensation in my chest was reduced, the feelings of anxiety before going to sleep ceased and I no longer felt so weakened. **Since mid-June (after only a month) there have been no angina pectoris symptoms, I can live without fear again and my quality of life has been very much improved.**

I can now live completely without complaints and without taking any medicines, which I very gradually reduced and later stopped taking altogether. My doctor found a distinct improvement so that the **balloon catheter treatment now no longer seems necessary.**

You can imagine how pleased I am!

Yours, in gratitude,

Hansjoachim Schmidt

Dear Dr. Rath,

Ladies and Gentlemen,

During a catheter examination in February this year the cardiologist found that an **80 percent constriction of the left coronary artery** (LAD) had **reduced to 50-60 percent** since May last year. This stenosis had not been dilated the previous year.

The doctors in attendance are aware of my participation in a vitamin program and that I am a student of Cellular Health. They agreed that they do not know of any other reason for the reduction in the stenoses. Your books and research made the difference.

Yours sincerely,

D.M.

Dear Dr. Rath,

Two years ago I suffered a **posterior wall cardiac infarction.** After my stay in the hospital and subsequent curative treatment, a two-vessel coronary disease was diagnosed at the subsequent cardiac catheter examination.

Following successful vascular dilatation by balloon catheter, new problems arose, in particular shortness of breath and faintness. Another opening of the vessels was refused, however. At the time I was very disappointed as I was now to live with a certain amount of risk.

Since February this year I have successfully been following a vitamin program after reading about the benefits of vitamins in your books. **I feel very much better today and the problems have all but disappeared.**

I should like to offer you my thanks and shall also tell others with the same complaints about my experience.

Best regards,

R.L.

Dear Dr. Rath,

I am **35 years old** and I have been suffering acutely from constriction of the coronary vessels for six months. In November 1997 I suddenly had a **heart attack with fibrillation and respiratory arrest. I had to be resuscitated,** had balloon catheter treatment and a Stent*. It was a real shock to suddenly almost die at my age.

I read your research and since February this year I have been taking supplements of vitamins and minerals. **After four weeks the cholesterol level has fallen and my energy has increased.** Even sports are possible again to a normal degree (ten years ago I was a professional soccer player!)

On 7th May this year I had another catheter examination: All blood vessels are open, blood results are good and I feel well.

I have told other patients of my experience with vitamins and wish them the same progress that I have had.

Yours sincerely,

Dieter Kurth

*Metal prosthesis mesh that is implanted into the arterial wall to prevent the vessel from closing up.

Dear Dr. Rath,

I am 68 years old and for eleven years I have been suffering from **angina pectoris with piercing pains** in the left upper arm with any kind of movement, with feelings of panic, and shortness of breath. Then I had a **heart attack**. The pressure pains, nausea, shortage of breath, and the fear were unbearable.

Since April this year I have been taking vitamins supplements and reading about Cellular Heath.

After three months there were no more pressure pains, no nausea, and no panic attacks. What is particularly encouraging to me is that I can again take long walks, carry my shopping bag myself, and tie my shoelaces without assistance. Inconceivable before!

Also I no longer need any Nitrospray and was able to cease taking other medicines. I am very grateful to you.

I probably don't need a bypass operation any more!

Yours sincerely,

Ingeburg Köhler

Dear Dr. Rath,

I heard and saw your video "The Chemnitz program" in July 1997 and read your book "Why Animals Don't Get Heart Attacks" with interest.

I am 60 years of age. Since childhood I have had severe attacks of migraine (twice to three times per week) and autonomic heart complaints since my youth. For about 20 years I have had **angina pectoris complaints, and high blood pressure with heart pains, rapid heart rate, pains extending to the shoulder and often to the hand**, swelling of the blood vessels on the left side of the neck, shortness of breath, and panic attacks.

Since August I have been on a vitamin regimen and feeling great.

Since then my health has improved markedly, with migraines only occurring seldom and mildly. **No heart complaints any more!**

In 1974 and 1986 I had varicose vein operations in both legs. Even afterwards I still had circulatory problems, heavy legs, pain, and agitation. These are now things of the past too!

I am very grateful to you and hope that you can help many other people.

All the best for you and your research!

Kind regards,

Crista Raderecht

Dear Dr. Rath,

In October I had my 84th birthday.

On January 31, 1991, it was very cold and I was out in the open. Suddenly severe pains shot through my chest and left arm. I went to the hospital in Gießen-- **heart attack.**

In the ensuing period I was plagued by **heart pain**, particularly when there was a change in the weather. In December 1997 I read your books and began a vitamin program to help my condition. **After three months I had no more heart pain** and no more sensitivity to changes in the weather.

I can drive a car and cycle again, work in the garden, and lift normal loads.

On July 16 this year I went for a check-up at the hospital. The ultrasound showed that the **calcium deposits** in the region of the left ventricle had been **reduced**. The doctor examining me was amazed at the improvement in my condition.

I am well!

Yours sincerely,

Ernst Grün

Dear Dr. Rath,

Today as a user of vitamins and a believer in Cellular Health, I would like to send you a report on my success.

I am 69 years old and have had **irregular rhythm of the heart (arrhythmia)** since 1983 and since then have had a pacemaker. On December 7th, 1996, I had a **heart attack**.

During the whole of last year I constantly had health problems and at least twice a month attacks of angina pectoris. My ability to cope was severely restricted. In November/December I suffered **extreme loss of energy** and constant heart pain. I could hardly raise my right arm due to the severe pain.

I was invited to see one of your lectures. Here I gained new hope. Since mid-December I have been taking nutritional supplements and cannot believe the difference they have made.

Christmas of last year I **no longer had severe pain.** In January I was almost without pain, my right arm had full movement again, and **my general well-being had drastically improved.**

In contrast to the previous year, my health is good to very good. **I can do the gardening again almost without restriction,** which was inconceivable in the fall of 1997. In summary I can say that that the hope I gained from your lecture has been substantiated. I would like to express my thanks for this.

Yours sincerely,

P.H.

Dear Dr. Rath,

I am 72 years old and have suffered from **angina pectoris** for three years, characterized by severe pain behind the breast bone. After angioplasty (vascular dilatation by means of a balloon catheter) a blood clot had formed. Consequently, a **bypass operation** was performed. Two years later, **I again suffered from pain and shortage of breath, even with very slight exertion.** I searched for a way my body could help itself. I found the books on Cellular Health.

Since May 13th this year, I have been taking vitamins and minerals. **After only two weeks I was more energetic and had no shortness of breath. The recurrent heart pains with panic attacks have completely gone**, thanks to Cellular Health.

I am already planning to give your book to my friends, relatives, and neighbors. **I want to help in the battle against death from heart disease, and I know how valuable health is.**

Yours sincerely,

H.A.

Dear Dr. Rath,

I am **34 years old** and have been suffering from circulation problems for seven years.

Physical exertion would cause nausea and even vomiting. Other attendant symptoms were cold, stiff hands, faintness, and circulatory collapse. Most of all I suffered from nausea and a feeling of a lack of oxygen.

A friend told me of your work and since January this year I have been taking a vitamin regimen.

After two months the attacks of nausea and vomiting completely ceased. I have a **much better capacity** for particular physical exercise, such as exercises to keep fit.

My quality of life has improved considerably due to taking the vitamins. I feel well and am happy to be able do something positive for my body. My thanks to Dr. Rath and his research team.

Yours sincerely,

Jim Mende

Dear Dr. Rath,

I am 64 years old and suffered a **heart attack** while in the best of health (slim, normal blood pressure, and 159 mg cholesterol), so it was without warning. **After the heart attack** I often suffered heart pain, even when at rest, also **tiredness** and **edema of the legs.**

Now, since discovering the breakthroughs of your research I have been taking vitamin supplements, I have **no more heart pain. The edemas in my legs have disappeared.** Above all the severe exhaustion I experienced during the day has disappeared.

But the most wonderful thing of all is that I need no longer be in constant fear of a second heart attack (which is mostly even more dangerous). Near to where I live, a man of 38 years of age died from the first heart attack and three men between 40 and 50 died of the second.

I am eternally grateful to you for your research. I really hope you win the Nobel Prize.

With best regards,

E.W.

Dear Dr. Rath,

I am 58 years old and for several years have been suffering from occasional **heart pain**. The pains in the left side of the chest periodically extending to the **left shoulder and left arm** were agonizing. Furthermore I often had problems with cold feet, influenza, and angina.

I discovered your books on Cellular Health and, I have been taking vitamins and other supplements since August of last year.

After three months I noticed a considerable improvement in my state of health and capabilities. Furthermore, I can rejoice in having **no more heart pain and no more cold feet.** Since August last year I have had no more troublesome infections.

In brief, I feel good about myself again! I am very grateful to you!

Yours sincerely,

Wilhelm Raderecht

Dear Dr. Rath,

I am 62 years old and for about ten years I have suffered from **tightness of the chest and respiratory problems.** The following symptoms caused me a lot of trouble: tightness of the chest, shortness of breath and wheezing noises when breathing (not asthma, according to the doctor).

Six years ago I had a **heart attack** with no warning. After the attack I suffered from **bouts of circulation problems, tight chest, difficulty breathing, high blood pressure (at times 210/100),** periods of going hot and cold (head hot, body cold), and panic attacks. I was found to have a high cholesterol level.

I had to be sent to the hospital by ambulance five more times (always in the evening or during the night).

Since October I have been taking vitamins and minerals. Your research led me to a natural way to wellness. It seemed like such a smart thing to do.

Soon I noticed an improvement in my health – actually, I have to say right away, for I had no more attacks. After five weeks my blood pressure was normal (first reading up to 160, second always below 90). I could walk uphill, which hadn't been possible for years. Life is again worth living.

I was able to cut my heart medicine dosage in half, although it took a lot to persuade the doctor.

At one consultation, the doctor said: "If I didn't know better I would say you are quite healthy."

Dear Dr. Rath, you are the best thing that's happened to me in my life so far. I now want to live another 100 years to the full. Thank you.

Yours sincerely,

Doris Schlier

P.S. **I have now discontinued all my medicines** (ASS 100 and Xanef). My blood is thinned by Vitamin C, Vitamin E, and beta-carotene. My high blood pressure was reduced long ago due to the vitamin program. I am well.

Dear Dr. Rath,

I am 59 years old and have been suffering from **heart and circulation problems** for three years. At the end of November 1995 I suffered **severe infarction of the anterior wall**. I had little chance of survival. There followed a rehabilitation period of seven weeks. During that time, I read your literature.

In March 1996 I began taking a vitamin program. Now after about 15 months **I notice an improvement in my general condition. I was able to reduce the amount of medicine I take, in consultation with my doctor. My blood pressure is stable.**

I learned about vitamins from the information in your book. It should be recommended to everyone, young people in particular!

My family and many of my friends use a vitamin program.

Yours sincerely,
Ulrich Plettendorf

Dear Dr. Rath,

I am 73 years old and for many years have had **circulatory problems**. Two years ago I had operations for **four bypasses**. Seven weeks later I had an operation to remove two-thirds of my stomach.

I was so weak that I could no longer drive, not to mention doing light jobs. My condition got worse and worse.

At the beginning of May this year I heard of Cellular Health. I started slowly with a multivitamin foundation and after four weeks also began taking other nutrients. Now, after only six weeks, I feel much better, am driving again, and can help my wife with the housework.

We are both so happy and my wife has now also begun a vitamin program.

We thank you very much and hope that you can help many more people.

Yours sincerely,

K.H.M.

Dear Dr. Rath,

I am 63 years old and have suffered with heart problems for 12 years. I already had **two heart attacks and a bypass operation**. Three other arteries had already closed up again and were, I was told, inoperable as they were in a dangerous place.

In particular I suffered from **severe breathing difficulty, heart pain, and feelings of oppression**, which led to repeated ambulance trips to the hospital. As a result of being in the hospital and in my weakened condition, I was almost helpless and unable to do the housework. My neighbor had your book on Cellular Health and thought it could help.

Since April last year I have been taking a vitamin and mineral regimen. **After only several weeks I was much better, and in the meanwhile the heart pains and breathing difficulties with panic attacks have almost completely gone.**

I am so well that I can again do all my work in the house and even some work outside. I am so happy with this improvement!

Already six of my friends are taking vitamins. I would like to thank you for your research.

Yours sincerely,

I.M.

Dear Dr. Rath,

Three years ago, at the age of 69, I suffered **infarction of the anterior wall**. After that, three dilatations were performed. At a subsequent cardiac catheter examination I was asked for my immediate consent to a bypass operation, which I did not give, however. And so I went home with mixed feelings.

I had resigned myself to the fact that I now had to go easier with everything. Walks were limited; **even at the slightest incline I had to stop and take a deep breath.** There was also a feeling of uncertainty, accompanied by mild faintness. Intensive physical activity exhausted me and brought me out in sweat. I also began to suffer from increased sensitivity to changes in the weather.

After hearing about ypur work, I did my own research and I have been taking a vitamin regimen now for eight weeks. **My general condition has considerably improved in this period.** I can take longer walks in the forest again along the same routes that exhausted me before, or which I couldn't manage after the heart attack.

The feelings of uncertainty and faintness have completely gone too. I no longer need the strong cardiac stimulants.

Your research work is a blessing for me – and I hope for many others too. Thank you very much.

Yours sincerely,

Elli Meschkat

Dear Dr. Rath,

First of all I would like to explain my original situation: I am approx. 22 kg overweight. In December of 1990 **I had a heart attack at the age of 44**. After an appropriate length of stay in hospital and subsequent rehabilitation treatment, I was still classified by the doctors as severely "at risk from heart attack" and I was constantly given pharmaceutical preparations. This was mainly treatment in the form of **tablets to lower my blood pressure, level of blood fats, and uric acid level (gout), and anticoagulants**. As a result of taking the medicines there was in fact no further heart attack, but the curative effect was negligible.

My physical condition was poor, I was susceptible to other illnesses, such as colds, and often had pains in the chest.

Results of your research gave me hope and since January this year I have been adding vitamins and nutrients to my diet. **From March on things began to improve. My blood pressure, (initial reading 180/110 despite blood pressure tablets) dropped to the normal level of 140/90. I have completely stopped taking the pharmaceutical treatment for levels of blood fat and uric acid and anticoagulants.**

In 1996 I also developed diabetes. With a blood sugar level of 14 (250 mg/dl) I took one prescribed tablet per day, yet my sugar level remained just as high.

When I took the vitamins the sugar level fell to 7.0 (125 mg/dl). I intend, in consultation with my doctor, to stop taking the diabetes tablets as quickly as possible.

Since taking vitamins my physical condition is much improved. I am considerably stronger. I notice this when climbing stairs, cycling, at work and when working in the garden and in the house.

As a "side effect" of taking vitamins, I have become resistant to colds.

I would like to thank you. I consider myself fortunate to have found out about your research in the field of Cellular Health. I am convinced that the new ways of eradicating the "diseases of affluence" will be recognized.

I assure you of my full support in the battle against restrictive politics and the capitalistic interests of the pharmaceutical industry.

I wish you much success in your research.

Kind regards,

Christian Stoll

Dear Dr. Rath,

I am 52 years old and for eight years have suffered from **coronary heart disease with chest pain, tiredness, difficulty breathing, and stress problems** – in a word, angina pectoris.

In 1993 I learned of your work and I have been taking vitamins and minerals. After only four weeks my condition had improved.

I had balloon catheter treatment in 1991. As a checkup, this year I had a cardiac catheter examination. Diagnosis: excellent condition of the dilated vessel. **The coronary deposits have reduced since my taking of the course of vitamins.**

Yours sincerely,

K.K.

Appendix: Pictures of the cardiac catheter examination

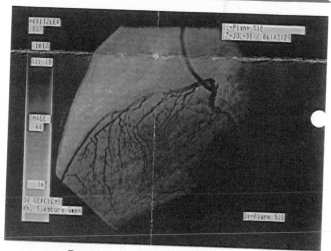

Contrast medium photo of the left
coronary artery dated July 17th 1991

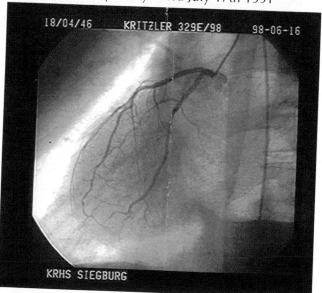

Follow-up picture of the left coronary
artery dated July 16th 1998

Dear Dr. Rath,

I am 65 years old. **For 17 years now I have been suffering from coronary vascular constriction and particularly pressure and tightness in the region of the heart and spasmodic pains. The medicine prescribed did not help.**

I read all your books from cover to cover and since April last year I have been taking vitamins and minerals added to my diet.

My heart rate stabilized and was markedly stronger after only one week. The above-mentioned complaints have almost completely gone.

I am very grateful for the help Cellular Health gave me.

Yours sincerely,

Ilse Karig

Dear Dr. Rath,

I am 77 years old and in 1982 had an **infarction of the posterior wall**. Also, my **left carotid artery was 50-60% closed, leading to dizziness and other problems.**

With the confidence inspired by your research I have been taking a vitamin regimen for about one and a half years regularly, three to four tablets a day. **Meanwhile, I am almost free of almost all the above-mentioned complaints!**

As long as I live I do not wish to be without the benefits of Cellular Health. My wife, (71 years old) is equally very pleased with the capsules she takes.

Yours sincerely,

H.J.

Dear Dr. Rath,

The state of my health has been characterized by a **heart attack** and severe **atherosclerosis,** which have already required four operations.

Now, after reading your books and taking vitamins for quite a long time, I feel considerably healthier. **All test results for risk factors, including cholesterol, have considerably improved** and I can definitely say I am in the "healthy" category.

Yours sincerely,

Johannes Michel

Dear Dr. Rath,

I am 59 years old and **for 24 years have been suffering from abnormal heart rhythm, high blood pressure, breathing difficulties, and pains in the chest.**

Then I heard your lecture and read your findings on Cellular Health. Since February this year I have been on a program that supplements my diet with vitamins and other nutrients. After six months I noticed that **my heartbeat was normal and my blood pressure had normalized from 200/100 to 140/80. What is particularly welcome is the fact that I hardly ever have pains in the chest.**

Finally, I would like to point out that I was earmarked for a **bypass operation**. That has been **postponed indefinitely.**

Yours sincerely,

R.H.

Dear Dr. Rath,

This letter is intended to give an insight into our success with Cellular Health.

Five years ago my husband, 90 years of age, was diagnosed as having **angina pectoris**. He had difficulty walking. After about 100 m he had **tightness of the chest and breathing difficulties.** The next step was always the **nitrolingual spray** which brought him temporary relief.

By chance we heard of your books, which gave us a lot of information. We acted promptly and immediately began a program to add vitamins and minerals to our daily diets. **Three weeks later there was improvement. After a further two months my husband again is able to walk greater distances without having to fall back on the nitrolingual spray. So, no more breathing difficulties and tight chest. Even his general condition has considerably improved.**

And now my own case: I am 80 years of age. Nine years ago I had a bowel operation (carcinoma of the colon) with subsequent chemotherapy. Since then I suffered from diarrhea, which was very unpleasant, and I could hardly undertake anything at all. All those medicines didn't help at all!

Then I thought, what helped my husband could also help me which is what actually happened. After two months I noted an improvement and two months later I was rid of that terrible malady. Therefore the basic vitamin program also helped in my case.

We began on May 15th last year and continue to this day. It gives me pleasure to tell you all this, Dr. Rath.

Now we hope and trust that the Cellular Health program will soon be available to the general public.

Yours respectfully,

Mr. and Mrs. K.

Dear Dr. Rath,

For 30 years I have suffered from **angina pectoris**. Now I am 60 years of age and on December 20th 1996, I had to undergo a cancer operation, followed by chemotherapy six times and tele-cobalt radiation 28 times. During and after this therapy I had more intense heart and circulation problems and low or severely fluctuating blood pressure.

Furthermore, I suffer from a congenital disease of the spinal column.

Then I heard about Cellular Health from a friend and decided to provide my body with vitamins. On April 2nd this year I began a thorough program.

The result: **I was able to stop taking the medicine for circulatory disorders in July.** In addition, I had severe stomach pains from years of taking medicine for my spine. I was able to discontinue this medicine too. What was amazing was that my spine problems did not get worse as a result. That was never the case before!

And so I had the courage to go mountain climbing; I walked or climbed to five mountain huts near Oberstorf/Oberallgäu (altitude 1800 to 2000m above sea level) in July of this year and was awarded the Oberstorf gold medal for climbing.

In contrast to the earlier period, when I always experienced pain in the region of the heart on inclines, I now had no problems.

I can only thank God for my good health, for his loving guidance allowed me to hear about the results of your research. In the meantime, I have already been able to recommend vitamins to many friends and acquaintances.

I thank you and wish you continued success and creativity.

Yours sincerely,

Regina Hübner

Dear Dr. Rath,

I am 47 years old. Three years ago I was diagnosed as having a **neglected anterior wall infarction (infarction of the anterior wall of the heart)**. The veins were blocked. I suffered from tiredness and weakness. In addition there were heart pains, which I tried to ignore.

A good friend told me of Cellular Health. Your research was hard to deny, and I have been taking vitamins and minerals since the beginning of March this year. Six months later an ultrasound scan showed that a **blood clot**, of which I had not been informed, had **completely dissolved.**

Yours sincerely,

W.U.

Dear Dr. Rath,

I am 78 years old and suffer from the following: severe asthma, auditory collapse, cancer of the prostate, and constricted veins supplied with blood up to only 30% in three places and up to 50% in five places. **Every 14 days I had severe heart attacks and had to go into the hospital.** I had to take 24 medicines at intervals throughout the day.

I was made aware of Cellular Health by my daughter. Since the end of January 1998 I have been taking vitamins twice a day. I wanted to stop after a week as I had pains in various places. I was advised to continue as it was probably a symptom of detoxification. I continued to take the formulas regularly.

It was good that I did! Today I can say that I am much better! No severe heart attacks any longer, no hospitalization!

My doctor is also working with Cellular Health. I pass it on wherever I am.

Thank you for your help.

Yours sincerely,

H. Adler

Dear Dr. Rath,

I am 66 years old and had a **heart attack** a year ago. **My capacity has been severely restricted ever since.**

Since May this year I have been taking vitamins three times a day as the result of reading your literature. After only eight weeks my condition was already considerably improved. **I can again walk for several miles without complaint and climb moderate hills.**

When I was re-examined by my doctor, he found that the irregularities in my heartbeat have also been reduced.

I can very much recommend vitamins to anyone.

Yours sincerely,

Gerhard Hohmann

Dear Dr. Rath,

Thanks to my children I heard of the success of your research work and read the book "Why Animals Don't Get Heart Attacks But People Do." For years I suffered from **angina pectoris and had to be repeatedly taken to the hospital with severe heart attacks.** Panic attacks, breathing difficulties, and pain characterized my state of health. Even short walks were difficult. Despite the doctors' efforts there was hardly any progress. I had to use nitrolingual spray several times a day, which brought only brief relief.

Since September last year I have been following a vitamin regimen. After only five to six weeks my condition was markedly improved. **I feel well all round and I am happy again.**

A few days ago I had a long-cherished wish fulfilled. I flew to Tenerife with my children and celebrated my 81st birthday there. **Without health problems, I am free of pain.** Thank you very much. I wish you strength and success in your work.

Yours sincerely,

E.R.

Dear Dr. Rath,

I am 58 years old and for a year I have suffered from **coronary disease** with severe stenosis (vascular constriction) that manifests itself as **painful throbbing in the chest** and simultaneous **breathing difficulties**, even with slight exertion. Most of all I suffered as a result of the medicines I had to take after a balloon catheter operation.

I heard that vitamins could help and read your books. Since May 19th this year I have been taking vitamins and other nutritional supplements. **The throbbing in the chest region subsided and I was again able to do my housework alone. After only three days this leaden tiredness disappeared.**

My doctor saw the good results from the vitamin program and helped me to discontinue my medicines gradually. My skin problems also slowly subsided.

Yours sincerely,

G.A.

"Functional" Heart Complaints
Dr. Rath's Cellular Health for
Prevention and Health Maintenance"

In many cases, heart problems such as pressure in the chest and rapid heart rate occur without any constriction of the coronary arteries.

In contrast to angina pectoris, the tight chest occurring predominantly during physical exercise can happen without any identifiable cause. These complaints are therefore called "functional," which is equal to "cause unknown."

Until now, medicine was unaware of any treatment for these heart complaints that were so unpleasant for the patients. Out of ignorance, medicine christened these complaints "heart neuroses" and the doctors prescribed psychiatric drugs, which often made the patients even more ill.

The following patients' reports document that even the principal cause of "functional" heart complaints is a lack of vitamins and other cell factors. Therefore even this common disorder has become causally treatable and will be largely unknown in the future.

Dear Dr. Rath,

I am 49 years old and have been suffering since May last year from **functional heart problems.** They are triggered by sudden panic and develop into **high blood pressure, rapid heart rate, and symptoms similar to a heart attack.**

Since May this year I have been taking vitamins and minerals and other nutritional supplements and **noticed after only a month that the anxiety attacks had considerably reduced.** When they do still occur, my pulse and blood pressure remain constant. **I stopped taking beta-blockers and psychiatric drugs. My whole condition has improved**. I would not like to be without the vitamin tablets any more. A year of "anxiety" combined with many stays in hospital is now a thing of the past since June 1998.

With the help of your research, I came across the vitamin program as I worked by myself to try to understand my illness, and I noticed from my own study that **disorders of a psychosomatic nature are often triggered off by stress**, but stress is a "robber of vitamins" I thought, as a "heart patient," a prophylactic with a vitamin program could do no harm.

The result is that I am now again free from symptoms. You have the answer to good health. More people should listen.

Yours sincerely,

Dietmar T. Holtwiesche

Dear Dr. Rath,

I am 61 years old and since the birth of our three children (1960-1962), I have suffered **heart problems, stabbing pains in the chest, and aching in my left arm. All the ECGs hitherto showed nothing, under exertion or relaxed**. On checking my pulse during senior citizen keep fit exercises, I noted irregularities. Otherwise, in **stressful situations**, I suffer from the complaints described above, and also from tiredness and loss of energy. Then I learned about Cellular Health.

Since April 20th this year I have been following a comprehensive vitamin regime **After taking the vitamins for ten weeks, my physical and mental efficiency had markedly improved**. My lipoprotein (a) level improved from 40.5 mg/dl (on 27.3 this year) to 28.5 mg/dl (on 23.6).

Yours sincerely,

H.D.

Dear Dr. Rath,

I am now 45 years old and for about six years   I have suffered from **circulation problems and indefinable heart pain**. This pain is accompanied by a great inner restlessness and aching in the left arm. Most of all I suffered from **constant pains in the region of the heart. Troubled sleep** was associated with this and, hence tiredness and bad temper during the day. Also, I noticed a swelling of the legs and ankles in the evening. Despite all my efforts (relaxation training, extended walks, etc.) there was no improvement.

From the April 1st of this year I have taken vitamins and worked for cellular health. Your books really helped.

Three weeks after I started the vitamins, I was pleased to notice that **the pain in the heart region had considerably reduced** and I was able to sleep peacefully. In the following weeks the heart pain almost completely disappeared and I again had **the feeling of well-being I had lacked for so long.**

-2-

The swelling in my ankles was much less. Also other problems, such as numb hands and cramps in the legs, only occur very rarely. You can imagine how pleased I am about this.

Of course, I have told my GP about it and the referral to a heart specialist is now unnecessary.

I wish to thank Dr. Rath and his people from the bottom of my heart as it is simply wonderful to feel so healthy and well again.

I shall take pleasure in passing on reports of my good experience and this letter, whose publication I fully support, would be an opportunity for that.

Yours sincerely,

Birgid Frei

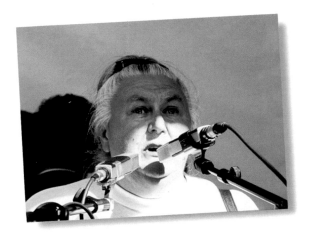

**Another patient who refused
"the business with disease".**

2

Stroke and Circulatory Problems in the Limbs

Studies show that circulatory problems of the brain, legs, and other organs and parts of the body are caused by calcification of the arteries (atherosclerosis), the same as circulatory disorders in the heart.

The following patients' reports of success indicate that circulatory problems can be almost as much a thing of the past as heart attack, stroke, leg amputation, and others.

**Cellular Health
for Natural Prevention
and Health Maintenance**

Dear Dr. Rath,

I am 79 years old and in August 1997 had a **first stroke** and in December 1997 a **second**. The resultant damage was **hemiplegia** in addition to **paralysis of the organs required for swallowing and speech**, and therefore I needed a special diet.

Since March this year I have been taking vitamins and minerals. After about ten weeks t**he difficulties in swallowing subsided; I can eat again, say a few words, and I can walk again. The research you published convinced me of the value of proper nutrition.**

I informed my doctor of this improvement and she was able to confirm it. I currently only have a special diet as a snack. My mental health has improved and **after three months of further supplements my blood sugar has fallen from 12 (215 mg/dl) to 6 (108 mg/dl).**

Yours sincerely,

Anna Wöhner

Dear Dr. Rath,

I am 36 years old and for six years have been suffering from constriction of the **carotid arteries (intracranial stenoses of the arteria cerebri anterior and the right media)** in addition to an excessive enlargement of the cranial artery (basilar cranial aneurysm). **The disease caused the following complaints: symptoms of paralysis in the left side of the body, no strength in the left side, fainting, and speech difficulties.** Most of all I suffered from the fact that I couldn't learn and understand anything new and also from a feeling of helplessness. A friend told me of Cellular Health and read your books to me.

I have been following an encompassing vitamin program since the May 29th this year. I have noticed the following improvements after two months.

My left arm has no **paraesthesiae (abnormal sensations caused by circulation disorders in the brain), my memory is better, I am more energetic, I can again hold objects in my left hand, and I can open bottle tops.**

I informed my doctor of this improvement in my health and he was able to confirm that my general condition and blood count are good.

Yours sincerely,

S.H.

Dear Dr. Rath,

A friend of my wife brought us your program "Fight Death from Heart Disease." After reading your brochures and hearing your audiocassette I bought your book "Why Animals Don't Get Heart Attacks." That was at the beginning of this year. In the meantime I am inspired by your research into cellular health!

On July 28th 1996, while at work I had a cerebral infarction as the result of a **vascular occlusion in the brain**. "You were lucky, because the adjacent regions continue to supply blood via the fine capillaries of this area," said the senior hospital physician.

I did well after my stay in hospital. I showed no signs of paralysis. I only experienced fainting attacks, which were twice very strong during the infusion period. Today I still have to take the medicines prescribed by the hospital! Why, actually?

As improving the vascular system was paramount to myself and my wife, starting a vitamin program seemed reasonable.

After a month of adding vitamins and other nutrients to my diet, **my general condition has improved, and difficulty breathing when climbing stairs or walking in the mountains has disappeared. I only rarely feel dizzy.**

I have already told many acquaintances, friends, and neighbors about the power of vitamins.

Thank you, Dr. Rath, for your important research, which must benefit everyone and is affordable!

Yours sincerely,

Christoph Weigert

Dear Dr. Rath,

I am already having great success with Cellular Health and I am impressed by your research. In the case of my mother, who suffered **two strokes**, part of her speech was affected by the second. Since then she has been totally pumped full of medicines and infusions to thin her blood.

After some persuasion, I was able to talk my mother into also taking a vitamin regimen. She has now been taking the vitamin tablets (3x2) **for over a year with success and her speech is as good as new (apart from a few irregularities that remain).**

I not only attribute that to the medical treatment but also clearly to the vitamin supplement. For this reason I fully support your program.

I remain,

Yours sincerely,

J.S.

Dear Dr. Rath,

I am 65 years old and for ten years I have suffered with **severe circulation problems. I had constant pain in my legs** and there was **no blood supply in my big toes.** Walking was sheer agony for me. I stumbled onto your research and was fascinated.

In October last year I began taking a program with vitamins and minerals. **After four months I could move my toes again! The pain was drastically reduced. I feel better month by month.**

Indeed, I feel so well that in May this year I even painted my niece's house. Up the ladder, down the ladder!

Six months ago I could hardly walk without a cane.

Furthermore I had to take tablets for irregular cardiac rhythm and for high blood pressure for ten years. Three months ago I was able to discontinue both medicines.

I don't see a doctor these days.

The vitamin program has improved my quality of life so much that I would like to thank you from the bottom of my heart.

Yours sincerely,

Bruno Randszus

Dear Dr. Rath,

I am 53 years old and for 15 years I have had **problems with circulation in my legs**. This manifested itself in that I had severe pains in my calves, particularly in the evenings. My uncle had good luck with vitamins and encouraged me to try them. I learned about Cellular Health and believed vitamins could help me.

Since May 15th of this year I have been taking vitamins and minerals. **After two weeks the pain in my legs was only slight, and after three months the symptoms had disappeared without a trace!**

I am an adviser in your network and have had only good experiences! Thank God for vitamins!

Yours sincerely,

Josef Kohler

Dear Dr. Rath,

Today I want to say thank you. I have been taking vitamins and nutritional supplements for about two months.

I have to say I was extremely skeptical but the research in your books seemed accurate. Somehow I expected overnight success in my condition. This was not immediately the case, until I suddenly noticed that the **circulatory problems in my legs had gone.**

I now again feel life in my legs. It's a completely new sensation, **to be able to stand and walk without difficulty**. All year I had been afraid of sunny days because then it was much worse.

So vitamins gave me a new start and I am now confident that everything else will go well.

Yours sincerely,

Maria Gröger

Dear Dr. Rath,

Today I can describe the first success of using vitamins and minerals

I have to say I am impressed by the results of your research and the Cellular Health program. I had always hoped for really effective means to tackle the problems at the root in a natural way. I immediately gave it my full attention.

I am 57 years old, tall and slim and have always tried to eat healthily. Despite my efforts in this regard, I developed **problems in the region of my left thigh: protruding veins,** "spider bursts," sensation of pressure accompanied by a nasty i**tching, swellings over the ankle** and as a result, **socks cutting into the flesh, and cold feet.** All this particularly occurred in the evening when my cold feet always prevented me from sleeping.

After about three weeks of taking the supplements, the itching and swelling have disappeared. The feeling of pressure has lessened considerably.

Finally I would like to express my gratitude and wish you every success in broadcasting the information about the Cellular Health Program, to which I am trying to contribute.

Yours sincerely,

Peter Chory

Dear Dr. Rath,

I am 42 years old and for five years have suffered from **circulation problems** that made me feel weak and tired. I constantly had **pain in my legs, shivering, lack of energy, and tiredness.** On getting up in the morning already I had no energy.

I have been taking a vitamin regimen for three months. **Six weeks after starting, I noticed that the circulation in my legs was better and I had no pain. I am generally fit and more energetic than ever before.** I am a living example of what Cellular Health can do.

There are no traces of lack of energy or tiredness. I now go through life with vigor.

I am happy that there are people like you who help mankind back to health using harmless vitamins.

Yours sincerely,

M.U.

Dear Dr. Rath,

I am 63 years old and for six years I have suffered from **circulation problems**, in particular **calcium deposits in the right carotid artery**. This condition often caused a **rushing noise in my right ear.** My cousin had your book that addressed my condition. I read it all one night.

Since the fall of 1996 I have been taking vitamins and minerals. After 18 months my circulation was tested and an EEG was performed by my neurologist.

The transformation was remarkable as the **arteries are completely clear again and the noise in my ear has disappeared.**

I am overjoyed.

Yours sincerely,

R.M.

Dear Dr. Rath,

I am 50 years old and for two years have suffered from **circulatory problems.** I had **no sensation in my fingers.** I heard of your books and read them.

Since April I have been taking vitamins and nutritional supplements. **After nine weeks I could feel my fingers again.**

I am very satisfied with the vitamin program. I feel very well.

Yours sincerely,

M.S.

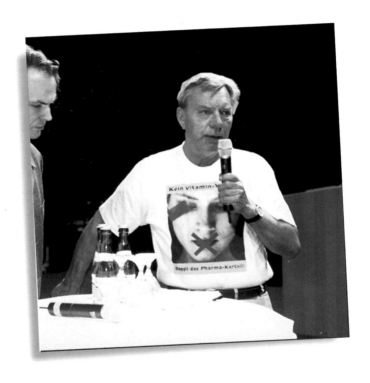

"If it weren't for vitamins and minerals, I wouldn't be here today."

3

Metabolic Disorders and Risk Factors

- **High Cholesterol Level**

- **High Triglyceride Level**

- **High Lipoprotein(a) Level**

**Cellular Health
for Natural Prevention
and Health Maintenance**

The Facts About Cholesterol and Other Secondary Risk Factors
Cholesterol Is Only A Secondary Risk Factor

Worldwide, hundreds of millions of people have elevated blood levels of cholesterol, triglycerides, LDL (low density lipoproteins), lipoprotein(a) and other risk factors. Contrary to what the pharmaceutical companies selling cholesterol-lowering drugs want to make you believe there is nothing wrong with cholesterol levels of 220 or 240. At best cholesterol is a secondary risk factor because the primary risk factor determining your cardiovascular status is the weakness and instability of your blood vessel walls. Elevated blood levels of cholesterol and other blood risk factors are not the cause of cardiovascular diseases but are the consequence of developing disease.

Conventional medicine is limited to treating the symptoms of secondary risk factors. Drugs blocking the synthesis of cholesterol and other lipid-lowering agents are now being prescribed to millions of people. These drugs are known to cause cancer and have other severe side effects. You should avoid them whenever you can.

Again, the reasons for elevated cholesterol levels are only partially understood by conventional medicine. Inherited disorders (genetic risk) and a high fat diet (dietary risk) are the two main reasons given in the textbooks of medicine. The most important reason is completely missing: a chronic deficiency of vitamins and other essential nutrients.

Modern Cellular Health provides a new understanding about the factors causing high blood levels of cholesterol and other secondary risk factors, as well as their natural prevention. Cholesterol, triglycerides, low density lipoproteins (LDL), lipoprotein(a) and other metabolic products are ideal repair factors, and their blood levels increase in response to a weakening of the artery walls. A chronic weakness of the blood vessel walls increases the demand for production of these repair molecules in the liver. An increased production of cholesterol and other repair factors in the liver increases the levels of these molecules in the bloodstream and over time renders them risk factors for cardiovascular disease. Thus, the primary measure for lowering cholesterol and other secondary risk factors in the bloodstream is to stabilize the artery walls and thereby lower the metabolic demand for increased production of these risk factors inside the body itself.

Therefore, it is not surprising that vitamins and other nutrients help in stabilizing the artery walls, and also, in parallel, help to decrease blood levels of cholesterol and other risk factors naturally.

My recommendations for people concerned with elevated cholesterol and other secondary risk factors. Lowering cholesterol without first stabilizing the artery walls is an insufficient and ill-fated cardiovascular therapy. Start as early as possible to increase the stability of your artery walls with essential nutrients to normalize blood levels of cholesterol and other risk factors.

Where there is vitamin deficiency, the liver receives the signal to increase production of repair factors to seal and stabilize the arterial wall

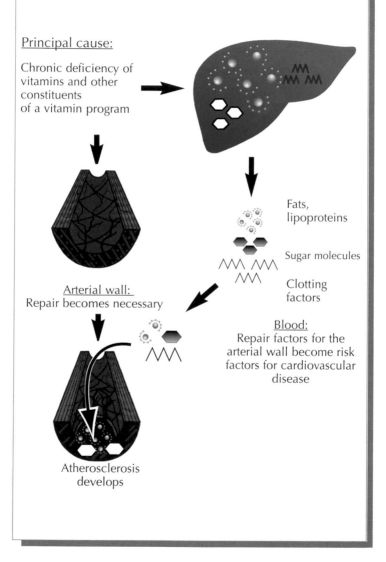

Principal cause:

Chronic deficiency of vitamins and other constituents of a vitamin program

Fats, lipoproteins

Sugar molecules

Clotting factors

Arterial wall:
Repair becomes necessary

Blood:
Repair factors for the arterial wall become risk factors for cardiovascular disease

Atherosclerosis develops

Dear Dr. Rath,

My first health check in 1995 (at barely 36 years of age) showed that my **blood cholesterol level was much too high** at 7.98 mmol/l (310 mg/dl). My doctor urged me to change my diet to low-fat food, which I did.

Nevertheless I was only able to show a **slight improvement at my annual check-ups**. The level was just low enough for me not to have to take any medicine. From 1996 to January this year the level was 6.60, 6.63, and 6.88 mmol/l (around 260 mg/dl). I was not able to reach the desired 5.7 mmol/l (220 mg/dl) so I had to have a check-up every four months.

At the end of the year, I read your books and vowed to change my life. At the beginning of this year I began a program with vitamins and minerals. Because of this program, the results of the cholesterol test on May 11th were **for the first time in the allowable range, i.e., 4.8 mmol/l (190 mg/dl).**

In addition, I feel much less susceptible to infection and this year avoided the cold and occasional bronchitis I normally suffer in spring. I am convinced that this success is due to a sufficient supply of vitamins and shall continue to take the supplements daily.

Yours sincerely,

M.L.

Dear Dr. Rath,

I am 43 years old and for three years have suffered from **high levels of cholesterol and triglycerides.**

Since learning of Cellular Health from your books, I have been taking vitamins and minerals since April of this year.

The level of cholesterol fell from 264 mg/dl to 185 mg/dl and triglycerides from 246 mg/dl to 134 mg/dl in only three months.

I was not able to achieve this through diet alone. With the vitamin program it was no problem.

I am impressed!

Yours sincerely,

Karin Anger

The mmol-l-value must be multiplied by 40 to convert the blood cholesterol level from millimol per liter (mmol/l) to milligrams per deciliter (mg/dl).

Dear Dr. Rath,

I am 68 years old. I have suffered from **coronary vascular disease** since 1985. On January 22nd, 1988 I had to have a **triple aorto-coronary vein bypass operation.** On January 29th, 1989 another aorto-coronary bypass operation had to be performed due the unsuccessful bypass implant on the coronary sinus.

When I read your book "Why Animals Don't Get Heart Attacks," my wife and I began a vitamin program in March of last year.

I have noticed the following changes in my condition:

Risk factor **lipoprotein (a)**
Result on 13./17.2 last year: 151 mg/dl
Result on 20./21.1 this year: 96 mg/dl.

HDL cholesterol ("good" cholesterol)
Result on 13.2 last year: 35 mg/dl
Result on 7.9 this year: 57 mg/dl.

Yours sincerely,

E.K.

Dear Dr. Rath,

Before I began taking vitamins,my **cholesterol level was 320 mg/dl. Now it is 180 mg/dl.**

Furthermore, the **triglyceride level and HDL-to-LDL cholesterol balance is also normal. Above all my lipoprotein(a) level fell from 15 to 1 mg/dl.**

I will continue to take the vitamins for as long as I live.

Many thanks for your research into a natural way of reducing the risk for heart and circulation diseases. Your books led me to good health.

Yours sincerely,

M.R.

Dear Dr. Rath,

All the years at the office had finally caught up with me. I was **tired, gaining weight**, and a recent visit to the doctor had revealed that I was on the **verge of diabetes** and a candidate for **high blood pressure**. My doctor wanted to do further tests, but a business trip took me out of the country for a few weeks.

Upon my return, I had to see my doctor. He prescribed medications to control my cholesterol and lower my blood sugar. I took the medicines but had bad reactions. My stomach did flip-flops and strange spots appeared before my eyes.

I took it upon myself to do research and find a way to make myself healthy. A friend referred me to your work, and I began including vitamins and minerals in my diet. After two months of taking the supplements, my doctor checked me and was amazed. All my levels had dropped to near normal, and had to agree that the natural methods were working. I plan on continuing taking the vitamins and feeling the best I can.

Thanks to you and your research. I will be happy to pass along my experiences to anyone I meet.

Yours Sincerely,

F.P.

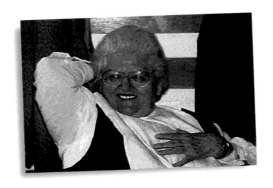

Maria Trapp can laugh again!

4

High Blood Pressure

**Cellular Health
for Natural Prevention
and Health Maintenance**

The Facts About High Blood Pressure

Worldwide several hundred million people suffer from high blood pressure conditions. The spread of this disease is largely due to the fact that, until now, the causes for high blood pressure have been insufficiently understood.

Conventional medicine concedes that the causes of high blood pressure are unknown in over 90% of patients. The frequent medical diagnosis, "essential hypertension" was established to describe the high blood pressure conditions in which the causes remain unknown. Accordingly, conventional medicine is confined to treating the symptoms of this disease. Betablockers, diuretics and other high blood pressure medications target the symptoms of high blood pressure, but not its underlying cause.

Modern Cellular Health provides a breakthrough in our understanding of the causes, prevention and adjunct therapy of high blood pressure conditions. The main cause of high blood pressure is a chronic deficiency of essential nutrients in millions of artery wall cells. Among other functions, these cells are responsible for the production of "relaxing factors" which decrease vascular wall tension and keep the blood pressure in a normal range. The natural amino acid arginine, vitamin C and other nutrients contribute to optimum availability of these artery wall relaxing factors. In contrast, chronic deficiency of these essential nutrients can result in spasms and thickening of the blood vessel walls, and can eventually elevate blood pressure.

The following letters from blood pressure patients vividly confirm this medical breakthrough. Cellular Medicine is now bringing an end to this endemic disease.

Cellular Health and High Blood Pressure

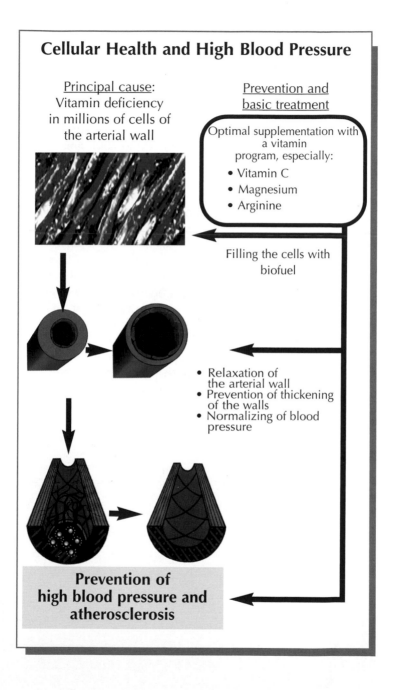

Principal cause:
Vitamin deficiency
in millions of cells of
the arterial wall

Prevention and
basic treatment

Optimal supplementation with
a vitamin
program, especially:
• Vitamin C
• Magnesium
• Arginine

Filling the cells with
biofuel

• Relaxation of
the arterial wall
• Prevention of thickening
of the walls
• Normalizing of blood
pressure

**Prevention of
high blood pressure and
atherosclerosis**

Dear Dr. Rath,

My aunt (age 70), had **severe problems with high blood pressure** (systolic values 180 to 200). **She could not tolerate the chemical antihypertensives due to the side effects.** She was quite desperate. I read your books and took vitamins and I therefore recommended to her a thorough vitamin program which she has now been taking for about four months. For one month she has also added other nutrients

The vitamin formula was effective and the upper value for blood pressure is on average 140 or 135, so has reduced considerably.

Her doctor looked at my aunt's chart and was very surprised and **pleased with the results** from taking the vitamin program. He immediately noted the address on the package.

Yours sincerely,

Arnold A. Neumann

Dear Dr. Rath,

I am **42 years old** and for two years have been suffering from **high blood pressure**. This condition, **at 150/100**, was treated with beta-blockers (atenolol 25). **Edemas (water accumulation) in my calves really got me down.**

Your research addressed my condition perfectly. In June of this year I began taking vitamins three times a day. After four weeks I tripled the quantity of this formula. **After seven weeks my blood pressure normalized at 130/90 and the edemas had noticeably reduced.**

Now neither beta-blockers nor other medicines are necessary.

Yours sincerely,

Harald Zastera

Dear Dr. Rath,

I am 48 years old and for three years have suffered from high blood pressure of 170 over 98. Most of all I suffered from **headaches** and **palpitations.** The doctor prescribed Xanef 5 mg twice daily.

Your research seemed compelling and for two months I have been taking a vitamin regimen. **My blood pressure is now 130 over 80. Wonderful!**

I no longer get headaches and my heart is now much more regular. There is no unpleasant palpitation. Also, I have noticed better circulation in my whole body and head. I can concentrate better, and I am better able to deal with stress. **In short, my general state of health has improved considerably.**

I shall continue to take the vitamin treatment as I have as yet found no doctor who can really help me.

Yours gratefully,

Anna Szczepaniak

Dear Dr. Rath,

I am 59 years old and for 18 years have suffered from **high blood pressure** with attacks of nervousness and dizziness. **Sexual inadequacy** has also troubled me greatly for three years. I was devastated. My wife threatened to take a young lover. The medicines prescribed by the urologist did not help at all. In February this year I read your books and began taking vitamins and minerals. **My blood pressure changed after only nine weeks from 200/110 to 145/90. My love life is also a success again. My wife only smiles now.**

Yours sincerely,

Manfred Szanzeitat

Dear Dr. Rath,

I am 61 years old and for 17 years have suffered from **high blood pressure. Dizziness** and **headaches** were the troublesome accompanying symptoms. My **blood pressure was 160/100.**

Since January of this year, I began vitamins and nutritional supplements, following the path you suggest in your books.

Now after six months I feel considerably better and my blood pressure has dropped to 132/72. I now only take half a tablet for blood pressure and hope to discontinue this soon.

I am very grateful to you and will continue to recommend vitamins.

Yours sincerely,

E.S.

Dear Dr. Rath,

I am 55 years old and **for 30 years have suffered from hypertension** (high blood pressure) and varicose veins. For years the high blood pressure was treated with medicines. In January this year I was admitted to the hospital with **hypertension and thrombosis, my blood pressure at 230/130**. I also suffered a lot from swollen legs.

Having studied your literature in May, I began a vitamin and mineral regimen. **After about eight weeks my blood pressure stabilized to 130-140/85-90.**

I was able to stop taking all but one of the medicines. I have no more problems with my legs and my varicose veins are not so severe as before.

I feel well again through vitamins and Cellular Health and can enjoy my professional life once more.

Yours sincerely,

R.S.

Dear Dr. Rath,

I have been taking **vitamins for nine weeks due to slight hypertension** (high blood pressure). I am 68 years old and **have already achieved normal blood pressure.** I am currently aspiring to the optimal 139/83 obtained in the HOT study.

In the last few days I have been able to cut the dosage of my ACE inhibitor (Lisinoporil) in half without my blood pressure increasing. With the reduction of ACE inhibitors several unpleasant side effects in my stomach and intestine also disappeared.

What prompted this experiment was the clinical study recorded at the end of the book "Why Animals Don't Get Heart Attacks" and the results mentioned there of the UCT (electron beam tomography) scan, which is sadly still not adequately available in Germany.

I have meanwhile been able to convince several friends to try a vitamin program and they are now too using it for their health.

I wish you every success in your work.

Yours sincerely,

Dieter Rehberg

Dear Dr. Rath,

I am 66 years old and for 15 years have suffered from **"essential high blood pressure"** with the following symptoms: shortness of breath, pressure in the region of the heart, feelings of stress, and uneasiness. My cholesterol level is also high.

Because of your research I have been taking vitamins and other supplements since March of this year.

After only six weeks my blood pressure was lower, there was no sign of the high-pressure period at midday, and in the evenings, in contrast to before, it only rose slightly.

Over time **my blood pressure returned to normal – despite cutting the beta-blocker medicine dosage in half.** Perhaps soon I won't need any beta-blockers at all any more.

I feel more active, younger. The vitamins noticeably heal the arteries and circulatory system bit by bit.

Yours sincerely,

I.L.

Dear Dr. Rath,

I am 78 years of age and have suffered from **high blood pressure** for 20 years. Also **cardiac insufficiency with water retention in the legs** and dizziness caused me a great deal of trouble.

I read your literature on Cellular Health and for four months I have been taking vitamins and other nutritional supplements in my diet.

After only four weeks my blood pressure fell – you can see this positive development yourself on the enclosed diagram.

The **water accumulation** in my legs has also reduced and I enjoy walks more again and **sleep better at night.**

My doctor has confirmed the improvements and consequently **discontinued the blood pressure medicine.**

My thanks to you and your team!

Yours sincerely,

I.L.

After 20 years of high blood pressure

Natural reduction in blood pressure
from 205/98 to 155/85 with
a comprehensive vitamin and
nutritional supplement program

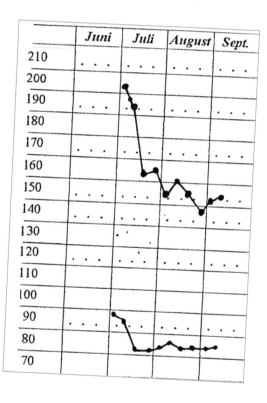

Dear Dr. Rath,

My blood pressure has been rather low all my life, then for the last few years I have suffered from **high blood pressure:** My legs, arms, and hands go numb.

The doctor treating me prescribed the beta-blocker Metoprolol retard–Ratiopharm (one 200mg tablet per day).

Then I read about Cellular Health and gave it a try. Since the beginning of May this year I have also been taking vitamins with my food.

Within 14 days the first reading of **my blood pressure dropped from 180 to 140;** it is currently 130! All the measurements were taken by my doctor.

Furthermore I can say that in addition, **my well-being and efficiency have been increased.**

I would like to thank you very much.

Yours sincerely,

E.H.

Dear Dr. Rath,

I have been a plasma donor for two years. Each time I donated, my blood pressure was taken. The results were recorded on a weekly basis (same day, same time).

I have become **concerned about my blood pressure results** as they were at the upper limit allowed for donating blood.

02.09.97	155/95
16.10.97	190/100
26.12.97	**165/90**

At the beginning of this year I learned of cellular health and began a vitamin program. My blood pressure has, to my delight, improved greatly since then.

10.04.98	130/85
02.07.98	140/80
12.08.98	**130/80**

I shall continue taking the vitamin tablets.

I am happy to s**upport your work that is so important for the health of mankind.** It feels good, too, to be able to help oneself and others.

I wish you every success in attaining your high objectives.

Yours sincerely,

R.E.

Dear Dr. Rath,

I am 67 years old and for seven years I have had problems with my circulation following inflammation of the cardiac muscle. I had **unstable blood pressure** constantly that fluctuated between normal and **high blood pressure.** My blood pressure has almost always been high since January. The winter gave me time to do research and I came across your Cellular Health books.

In June this year I began taking vitamins and other nutritional supplements. After only a month I noticed a relative s**tabilization of my blood pressure.** There was also an essential improvement in my well-being, and headaches were only infrequent.

I was able to stop taking "Isoket" and my blood pressure medicines.

Since the beginning of August this year I have taken additional nutrients for a few varicose veins needing treatment. I am confident here also.

Yours sincerely,

G.K.

Dear Dr. Rath,

I am 41 years old and for six years have suffered from **high blood pressure.** I had problems getting to sleep, insomnia, and weariness during the day. More than anything I suffered from severe palpitations when lying down and a pulse of 80 while at rest. A friend suggested that your books might help.

Since February of this year I have been taking vitamins and minerals. Before this, I had gradually stopped taking the prescribed beta-blockers*. After one day of severe withdrawal symptoms, everything normalized, even my pulse. After four weeks I had **no problems with stress** any longer.

I feel well and am happy to have found a solution to supply my body with the vitamins it needs in addition to healthy food and to be able to live without chemicals.

Yours sincerely,

E.B.

* Note: Please only reduce your heart medicines in consultation with your doctor.

Dear Dr. Rath,

I am 47 years old and have suffered from **high blood pressure** for ten years with the following symptoms: dizziness, tightness of the chest and tiredness, disturbance of the cardiac rhythm, and increased heart rate.

Since November of last year I have been taking a program of vitamins and minerals. After four months the tightness in the chest disappeared, the dizziness had gone, my efficiency had increased, and I can now get out of bed quickly in the morning.

The first reading of my blood pressure showed a fall from 180 to 135.

I have told my doctor about the Cellular Health program, but I got no reaction. His scepticism only subsided on seeing the good results.

By taking vitamins **I have discontinued my blood pressure medicine** and could present my doctor with the full proof.

The pharmaceutical prescriptions and their side effects did not help me. I wish your team continued success, and many thanks.

Yours sincerely,

A.H.

Dear Dr. Rath,

I am 52 years old and for 10 years have suffered from **high blood pressure** and **bleeding gums**. My blood pressure was 140/92 and my gums bled constantly when cleaning my teeth or eating an apple.

In April of this year I began taking vitamins and other supplements. after reading your books and deciding your suggestions could do no harm.

After eight weeks I had **no bleeding of the gums**, not even after vigorous brushing. Also, a medical check-up showed that my **blood pressure is now 120/80.**

Yours sincerely,

Hilmar Kickel

* Note: Hundreds of years ago, the first indication of vitamin deficiency in seafarers was bleeding of the gums.

Dear Dr. Rath,

I am a **high blood pressure patient**. Values of 160 over 100 were the order of the day and I was treated with medicines. As these resulted in a loss of drive, I simply stopped taking the blood pressure medicine. A check-up at the doctor's again showed excessive blood pressure, and I had to take medicines again.

It was a vicious circle, until one day, by chance, I saw the video of the "Chemnitz Program". Subsequently I read your book "Why Animals Don't Get Heart Attacks" and was introduced to the Cellular Health Program. I also began a regimen of vitamins and minerals.

After two months my blood pressure stabilized.

I stopped taking my blood pressure medicines bit by bit, and then completely. My blood pressure is now **completely normal at 140-146/86-88.**

I am impressed and at the same time convinced of the effectiveness of the vitamins.

After having such success myself, I passed your book on to a colleague. He also has problems with blood pressure and in addition the doctor has diagnosed **inflammation of the mucous gland.** He complained of **severe pains in the knee and had to be treated as an in-patient**. Since mid-December he has been taking vitamins and minerals and has been **free of pain and complaints since the end of February.**

With this account I would like to express our gratitude to you combined with the hope that you will provide us with yet more background information.

In this way we will be able to support your work towards building a new health care system to win the battle against death from heart disease.

Yours sincerely,

W.B.

Dear Dr. Rath,

Our mother has **suffered from high blood pressure for over 20 years.** Although she took antihypertensives as the result of two mild strokes, it was not possible to get her blood pressure under control.

Since May, on my advice, she has taken Coenzyme Q10, from July onwards a vitamin program and Depressan.

Now she only takes the vitamin program and follows your suggestion about Cellular Health, and no Depressan.

Everything has turned out well!

Thank you!

Christina Schönfelder

Dear Dr. Rath,

I have suffered from **high blood pressure** for five years and have to take medicines every day. I have been taking vitamins and minerals for five weeks now.

At the outset of the treatment, my blood pressure was **180/115;** after taking it for 14 days, it had fallen to 165/95 and the **last result was 130/80**. I attribute this improvement to taking the vitamins and what I learned from your books. I will continue to take them and will try to inform even more people about the health benefits of vitamins.

Yours Sincerely,

B.D.

Dear Dr. Rath,

I am 73 years old and **for seven years have suffered from high blood pressure.** This has already
been the cause of a heart attack. Furthermore I suffered a lot from tiredness, heart pain and dizziness.

I wanted to learn about nutrition and came across
your books. Since April 15th of this year I have been
taking vitamins and minerals.

After 19 weeks I noticed that **I no longer had
heart pain** when walking uphill, for example.

My blood pressure too had normalized and stabilized and my doctor advocates continued treatment
with the vitamin regime.

Yours sincerely,

A.O.

Dear Dr. Rath,

At the age of 37 I am suffering from **high blood pressure** and from cancer of the abdomen.

Cancer announced itself with extreme pains in the back and lower abdomen. I was plagued by the constant fear that this disease would spread.

Your research sounded good. I had nothing to lose. I have now been taking vitamins and minerals for the last three months.

After only two weeks my blood pressure normalized. I feel supremely well. My fear has subsided, because it feels good to know that my body is getting everything it needs.

I learned of cellular health from a friend. I will take the supplements for the rest of my life so that the cancer doesn't get another chance!

I have already and will in the future recommend vitamins everywhere; the effect was fantastic.

Yours sincerely,

Sonja Baggenstos

Dear Dr. Rath,

I am 51 years old and am writing this letter in gratitude for the help given to me by adding vitamins and minerals to my diet.

Ever since I was 28 I have had constant medical treatment for **high blood pressure**, angina pectoris and high cholesterol levels. Despite various medicines **my blood pressure was seldom below 150 /100.** There was no organic cause for my constant heart pain and increasing loss of performance.

Despite taking more and more different medicines to improve circulation and reduce blood pressure— beta-blockers to medicines to lower my cholesterol level—my condition continued to worsen. I had constantly swollen legs. I suffered increasingly from **tightness of the chest and difficulty breathing.** Worst of all was at night when I was awakened by **rapid heart rate.** During the day I was in constant fear from an impending heart attack.

Due to the inadequate curative effect of the medicines, I was given treatment for my complaints became increasingly expensive. For years I have been searching for other solutions or treatments that are more digestible or free from side effects. Increasingly I noticed the undesirable and harmful side effects of the drugs. Your books "No More Heart Attacks" and "Why Animals Don't Get Heart Attacks" clarified what I up to that point had only suspected or had not sufficiently understood about the connection between vitamins and health and the treatment of my illnesses.

I immediately stopped taking the medicines to lower my cholesterol level.

In December of last year I began a vitamin regimen.

The effect was amazing. After only two weeks of taking the vitamins, I felt noticeably better. After many years I could sleep through the night again. Two weeks later I was completely free of pain.

Since then my efficiency has also significantly improved. I do not tire so easily and can cope with stress again. **I can again go on strenuous walks and climb stairs without difficulty.** This was not the case before, despite taking medicines and various dietary supplements.

I am certain it was only the vitamin program and the unique combination of nutrients that made my rapid improvement possible. I am writing to you now, though I have been completely free of pain for several months. **I had to take medicines for more than 22 years, so I was afraid that the improvement without medicines might only be temporary**. I am convinced of the effectiveness of vitamins. Meanwhile I have been able to **discontinue taking all the medicines. My blood pressure is already 130/80 mm Hg. My cholesterol level is normal.** I feel very good generally.

I am happy that vitamins exists. Thank you for this.

Yours sincerely,

Udo Werner

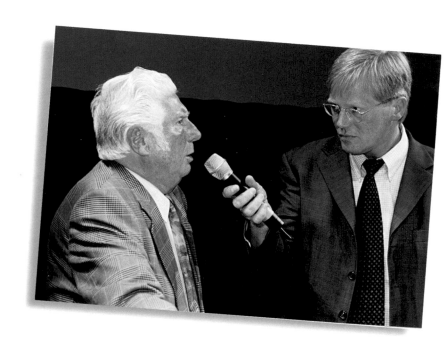

"No doubt Dr. Rath's findings will
transform modern medicine."

5

Heart Failure

- **Edema**
- **Shortness of Breath**
- **Fatigue**

**Cellular Health
for Natural Prevention
and Health Maintenance**

The Facts About Heart Failure

Tens of millions of people worldwide are currently suffering from heart failure, resulting in shortness of breath, edema, and fatigue. The number of heart failure patients has tripled over the last four decades. The epidemic spread of this disease is largely due to the fact that until now the causes of heart failure have been insufficiently understood, if at all. In some cases heart failure is the result of a heart attack; in most cases, however, such as cardiomyopathies, heart failure develops without any prior cardiac event.

Conventional medicine is largely confined to treating the symptoms of heart failure. Diuretic drugs flush out the water that is retained in the body because of the weak pumping function of the heart. Still, insufficient understanding of the causes of heart failure also explains the unfavorable prognosis of this disease. Five years after a heart failure condition is diagnosed, only 50% of the patients are alive. For many patients with heart failure, a heart transplant operation is the last resort. Most heart failure patients, however, die without ever having the option of such an operation.

Cellular Health provides a breakthrough in understanding of the causes, prevention, and adjunct treatment of heart failure. The primary cause of heart failure is a deficiency of vitamins and other essential nutrients that provide bioenergy to millions of heart muscle cells. These muscle cells are responsible for the contraction of the heart muscle and for optimum pumping of blood for circulation. Deficiencies of vitamins and other essential nutrients impair the pumping performance of the heart, resulting in shortness of breath, edema, and fatigue.

Cellular Health and Heart Failure

Principal cause:
Vitamin deficiency
in the millions of cells
of the heart muscle

Prevention and
basic treatment

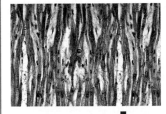

Optimal supplementation
with vitamins and
other nutrients:

- Vitamin C
- Coenzyme Q10
- Carnitine

Filling the cells
with bio-fuel

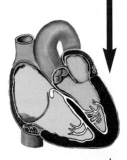

- Improved contractions
  of the cardiac muscle
  cells
- Increased pumping effi-
  ciency of the cardiac
  muscles
- Reduction of edemas
  and shortness of breath
- Improved physical per-
  formance

Prevention and
basic therapy for
heart failure

123

Dear Dr. Rath,

This letter should be considered a note of thanks. I can tell you that a vitamin program offers a good chance of survival.

As for me, I am 47 years old and have been **completely unable to work since my heart attack on March 29th, 1993,** since which time **I have hardly been able to undertake any physical activity.**

After the attack I was in the rehabilitation clinic and treatment with medication began. That went well until 1995, and then I took up smoking again. My body weight was mostly around 100 kg, and my height 1.71 m. So, I was constantly 30 kg over-weight. Further problems arose during January 1996, which I dismissed as side effects of the medicines and did not give too much thought to. Since this time, however, my efficiency and my quality of life had been severely restricted.

I tried to activate my body's own power to heal itself. I stopped taking my medicines without medical support. Things went relatively well until the end of the year, but then I suffered complete loss of strength. I had difficulty breathing and after two days I was admitted to the Marienhospital in Bonn on January 22nd with symptoms of decompensation of the left side of the heart. I was fitted with a pacemak-er. My heart was considerably enlarged.

After this the doctors told me that I must be prepared to have a heart transplant.

For final clarification I was transferred to the University Hospital in Bonn. The diagnosis was severe restriction of overall pumping efficiency, incipient arterial hypotension, coronary heart disease with 50% extensive stenosis (constriction), and thrombosis (blood clot) in the region of the right and left atria. On February 13th of this year I was discharged, continuing my treatment with Marcumar at home.

On February 18th I started taking steps towards rehabilitation. One of those steps was reading your books. Since then I have been taking a high dose vitamin program .

The check-up on March 5th showed a moderate reduction in heart size, **overall a significant improvement**. On March 24th, my heart size had again reduced and so, too, had the diameter of the central pulmonary arteries. On April 7th, again a significant reduction in heart size was recorded.

On April 29th I was admitted to the University Hospital in Bonn, as planned. No thrombosis could be found any longer in the right and left atria. I was finally discharged. **The transplant is no longer necessary!**

Since starting the vitamin program my physical performance has increased enormously and my quality of life is good again. I am convinced that the vitamin program has helped. I want to say a big "thank you."

Yours sincerely,

Lothar Meiszner

Dear Dr. Rath,

My mother has become increasingly weaker since mid-January this year. She could no longer get out of bed unaided, let alone get back in again. I had to feed her and sleep at her house to help her.

The GP diagnosed **cardiac insufficiency,** and the pumping efficiency got weaker and weaker.

As the **water accumulation in her feet** was getting worse, the GP changed the diuretic from "Disalunil" to "Furantil." My mother also had to take "Pholedrin longo" and "Myofedrin." My mother rapidly lost weight, five to seven kilos in a week, as a result of the **change in medicines**. Her feet were no longer swollen but instead she was totally **weakened**. I, by my own decision, stopped the tablets every four days. The **shortness of breath did not improve,** her blood pressure rose slightly to 100/70, and the weakness remained.

Since the beginning of May I have been giving my mother, now 93 years old, some vitamins and minerals in small doses.

-2-

Today we are amazed at my mother's recovery!

The shortness of breath is much better, the dizziness is gone, and likewise the water accumulation in her feet.

Her strength is slowly returning; she gets up herself and opens the door to receive visitors. **Her appetite has returned, and she no longer needs to be fed. Blood pressure is 120/80.**

All thanks to the Cellular Health Program!

My mother's state of health has considerably improved.

My mother and I would like to thank you, Dr. Rath, very much. Your research was not in vain. We are grateful that it is available to everyone.

Yours sincerely,

Else Weigert

Dear Dr. Rath,

My mother is 83 years old and for two years has suffered from cardiac insufficiency. She has already had two heart attacks. She suffers from **shortness of breath, accumulation of water in the lungs** and in the left leg, and tiredness. Shortness of breath was the worst thing for her.

She studied your research and since February this year she has been taking vitamins and minerals in moderate doses. **After only a week she noticed that the shortness of breath had considerably improved.** The diagnosed severe lack of white and red blood corpuscles and low hemoglobin level (also indications of anemia) had disappeared in two weeks. The planned spinal cord scan therefore did not take place.

Her heart has recovered well and her blood count is again normal. **It has been possible to reduce her heart medication and she was able to stop taking the diuretics completely.**

All in all we can say that my mother is doing well for her age, thanks to Dr. Rath's work.

Yours sincerely,

Anneliese Wallner

Dear Dr. Rath,

I am 53 years old and for two years have suffered from **cardiac insufficiency.** The effects were **shortness of breath, tiredness** and poor quality of sleep. Most of all I suffered from constant tiredness and the need to urinate during the night.

My aunt told me about Cellular Health and your work. For three months now I have been taking vitamins and minerals.

After eight weeks I noticed, for example, that **climbing stairs was not so difficult** and my quality of sleep had markedly improved. What was particularly welcome was that the **need to urinate during the night had reduced** and my efficiency during the day had improved.

An ECG confirmed the improvement in the action of my heart.

It was possible to reduce my dose of "Strophantin."

Yours sincerely,

M.M.

Dear Dr. Rath,

I am 71 years of age and **have suffered for ten years from cardiac insufficiency**. The complaints I suffered from were **difficulty breathing when climbing stairs, periods of exhaustion, and constant tiredness.** The most aggravating was the difficulty breathing after any exertion.

I heard of your research and wanted to try it for myself before taking prescription drugs. Since July 12th of this year I have been taking nutritional supplements, particularly vitamins and minerals.

After six and a half weeks I felt much stronger and even climbing stairs wasn't so much of a problem any more. My general condition has much improved.

Yours sincerely,

M.St.

Dear Dr. Rath,

I am a practitioner in alternative medicine and would like to tell you about a patient who has been using vitamin therapy as suggested in your books since July of this year.

The patient was diagnosed with arterial **hypertension (high blood pressure)** in 1980, and suffered an **anterior wall infarction** in 1996. Complaints since then have been **general debility, extreme tiredness, difficulty breathing, and faintness when climbing stairs.**

In March this year a deteriorated **insufficiency of the left side of the heart (cardiac insufficiency)** with critical hypertension and thrombosis (blood clot) in the left atrium, plus sclerosis of the aortic valve (calcareous deposits in the cardiac valve) were diagnosed. Since then, dizziness and unsteadiness when walking have presented themselves, as have continued tiredness and faintness. The patient takes the anticoagulant Marcumar.

At the end of July he began taking vitamin tablets (3x1).

After only ten days he no longer suffered from attacks of dizziness. After 25 days he reported climbing stairs is less strenuous and his customary after-lunch nap has been reduced from three-and a half hours to 1 hour.

The patient appears generally more alert. There have been **no more great fluctuations in blood pressure.**

The patient is now supplementing his diet further and feeling much better.

Yours sincerely,

I.S.

Dear Dr. Rath,

My husband has been suffering from cardiac insufficiency for several years. He was often in the hospital due to severe heart attacks and was treated with medication repeatedly—without success. My husband's stomach had a sensitivity reaction to the medicines so he ate less and less and lost weight.

About six weeks ago he was diagnosed with only 15% pumping efficiency of the cardiac muscle.

Our neighbor heard of my husband's plight and gave us your books. After my husband began a vitamin program, he improved from day to day. After only 14 days he could climb stairs again without having to stop on every second step. Even extended walks, which he had been unable to undertake for ages, are possible again.

We are so thankful to you, Dr. Rath, for this wonderful thing, and we tell all our relatives and friends about our experience with the power of vitamins.

Yours sincerely,

Cornelia Koth

Dear Dr. Rath,

I have been in the hospital twice already with **severe cardiac insufficiency**, the last time being this spring. I was discharged with several medicines, among them Marcumar.

A short time ago I learned of the Cellular Health Program from a newspaper article and requested extensive additional information from you. I immediately began a regimen to supplement my diet with vitamins and minerals.

First of all I began slowly, with a few vitamins in lower doses. Then I increased the dosage and felt the positive effects really quickly. The vitamins gave me **the vital push for more strength and pleasure in dealing with even extraordinary challenges and tasks.**

By supplementing with the vitamins and minerals and other nutrients, I have now been able to **reduce my heart medicine to a minimum and have stopped taking Marcumar completely.**

I am so pleased and thankful for this, and my husband and I will do all we can to support the use of vitamins.

Yours sincerely, and with best wishes for your courageous effort!

Maria Mühlmann

Dear Dr. Rath,

Eleven years ago I suffered a heart attack and had two bypasses. Despite the antihypertensives, my blood pressure systolic reading was all too often above 200 and was seldom below 180. Later shortness of breath was detected and the heart specialist prescribed ACE-inhibitors. Later still **cardiac insufficiency was diagnosed.**

I had never heard the words cardiac insufficiency before. **The build-up of blood in front of the left ventricle went as far back as the liver. For the next three years I only had a 50% chance of survival.**

The pumping efficiency was already so bad that a year ago I could only manage climbing a second step with panting, and four steps only with two pauses for rest.

On the other hand, I had to take Molsidomin three times a day. If I forgot to take even one tablet, one or two hours later I was vividly reminded of it by the tightness in my chest and difficulty breathing.

I hated the medication and found your literature. Two months after beginning a vitamin regimen, I was no longer aware of such reactions and stopped taking Molsidomin completely.

That means that only the vitamins have allowed the bioenergy to build up to improve my heart's pumping efficiency. Pharmaceutical prescriptions had made this impossible.

I found this very interesting, for since my heart attack, I have swallowed some 25,000 tablets. You cannot get healthy like that.

My thin waxy skin, which used to bleed easily, is back to normal again. **The agonizing daytime tiredness is gone. Also, I can now again climb up four steps like a healthy 66-year-old.** I went **uphill and downhill without complaint for two hours** on a school trip with my 9-year old granddaughter.

Also the medical examination showed that **my heart's pumping efficiency is better and my heart has decreased five centimetres in size. My blood pressure is now 125/75 to 140/85.**

I thank you, Dr. Rath, from the bottom of my heart. I expect to prolong my life now with your knowledge.

With best wishes to you and your team,

H.N.

Dear Dr. Rath,

I am 78 years old and for three years have suffered from **cardiac insufficiency** and circulatory problems. I was so weak that I could hardly walk.

My son had your literature and takes lots of vitamins. For three months, I have been taking vitamins and minerals.

I can say that I now feel much better. I can again do small jobs in the house. I can already walk short distances accompanied, which was not possible before.

I am very happy and grateful for this and hope I will continue to feel better.

Yours sincerely,

L.M.

Dear Dr. Rath,

I am severely restricted due to my weak heart.
Furthermore, I had to have surgery on both hands for
trapped nerves. Due to the fact that my GP recognized this too late, not only did my hands remain
without sensation but were also cold. I knew there
had to be a better way. I read all your books. Since
starting a vitamin program my hands are at least
warm again.

**I have been taking a varity of supplements and I
am better.**

Before, I had to lie down after 3-4 hours spent
upright (sitting or walking) due to my weak heart;
this is now only necessary after seven hours.

I can now also take longer walks. Previously I
could walk only 150 m; now I can walk 180 m. And
all that without the fear that it might harm me. I also
feel stronger.

I am 99 years old. This is confirmation of
Dr. Rath's results at any age!

Yours, in gratitude,

R.B.

Dear Dr. Rath,

I am 62 years old and for five years have suffered from arteriosclerosis with arrhythmia and angina pectoris, pains in the chest and shortness of breath.

After a severe heart attack my ability to endure stress was very severely limited and I suffered from constant tiredness and lack of energy.

I studied your research with the hope of feeling better and since mid-March I have been taking vitamins and other nutrients supplemented in my diet.

After only four weeks I noticed that my heart was beating more strongly, and that there was also no disturbance in cardiac rhythm nor angina pectoris pain. I was able to climb the stairs to my second floor flat quickly again and manage it without difficulty breathing, even with heavy bags.

At my ECG my doctor asked, what have they done to your heart?

Since the vitamin program I am a different person. I am simply happy! My energy has returned and I can take stress again.

Also the back pain that I had suffered for years has totally disappeared! It is simply wonderful!

Yours sincerely,

Gisela Hölzler

Dear Dr. Rath,

I am 42 years old and have suffered from a **weak heart** since childhood. This made itself apparent through **difficulty breathing during exercise**, such as climbing stairs, carrying heavy shopping bags and the like. I experienced an overall a chronic loss of strength. The constant lack of breath was the most unbearable part, however.

My mother gave me your books and since May this year I have been taking vitamins and minerals and supplementing my diet with other nutrients.

After eight weeks I was capable of much more. What was impressive was that I no longer need to stop when climbing stairs and my breathing normalizes really quickly.

In conclusion I would like to say that I previously had a severely enlarged heart and my muscles were weak too. I am sure that I can achieve a better quality of life through taking vitamins.

I hope you can help many other people with this.

Yours sincerely,

R.B.

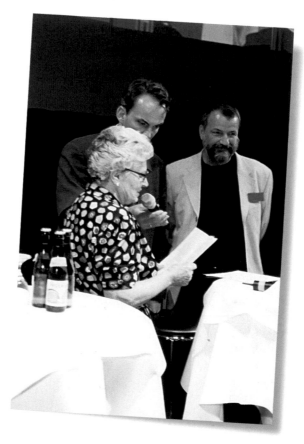

"Cellular Health changed my life!"

6

Irregular Heartbeat (Arrhythmia)

**Cellular Health
for Natural Prevention
and Health Maintenance**

Facts About Irregular Heartbeat

Over 100 million people worldwide suffer from an irregular heartbeat. Irregular heartbeat is caused by a disturbance in the creation or conduction of the electrical impulse responsible for a heartbeat. In some cases, these disturbances are caused by a damaged area of the heart muscle, e.g., after a heart attack. The textbooks of medicine, however, admit that the causes for most irregular heartbeat remain unknown.

Conventional medicine has invented its own diagnostic terms to mask its ignorange about most arrhythmias. "Paroxysmal" arrhythmia means "causes unknown." Consequently, the therapeutic options of conventional medicine can only treat the symptoms of irregular heartbeat. Beta-blockers, calcium antagonists, and other anti-arrhythmic drugs are given to patients in the hope that the incidents of irregular heartbeat decrease.

Charcterized by long pauses between heartbeats, arrhythmias are treated with a pacemaker. In other cases, heart muscle tissue that creates or conducts uncoordinated electrical impulses is cauterized (burned) and thereby eliminated. Lacking an understanding of the primary cause of irregular heartbeat, the therapeutic approaches by conventional medicine are unspecific and therefore frequently fail.

Modern Cellular Health now provides a decisive breakthrough in our understanding of the causes, prevention, and adjunct therapy of irregular heartbeat. The most frequent cause of irregular heartbeat is a chronic deficiency in vitamins and other essential nutrients in millions of electrical heart muscle cells. Long term, these deficiencies of essential nutrients directly cause, or aggravate, disturbances in the creation or conduction of the electrical impulses triggering the heartbeat. Thus, the primary method for preventing and correcting an irregular heartbeat is an optimum supply of vitamins and other essential nutrients.

Cellular Health and Irregular Heartbeat

<u>Principal cause:</u>
Vitamin deficiency
in the millions of cells
of the cardiac muscle

<u>Prevention and
basic treatment</u>

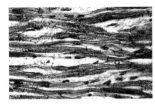

Optimal supplementation
with vitamins and other
nutrients:

- Vitamin C
- Magnesium
- Carnitine

Filling the cells
with bio-fuel

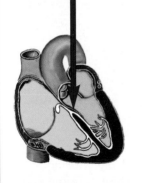

- Energy supply for
  electrical heart
  muscle cells
- Improved conduction
  of the stimuli respon-
  sible for heartbeat

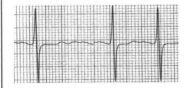

**Prevention and
basic therapy for
irregular heartbeat**

143

Dear Dr. Rath,

In 1992 I suffered a **heart attack (posterior wall)** and since then have had **insufficiency of the left side of the heart (weak pumping efficiency of the left ventricle).** In November of 1996 I chanced upon your book. Since my attack I had been studying specialized literature and also literature on dietetics. A change in diet brought mild relief from my complaints.

In the spring of 1995 I developed heart rhythm disturbance, which was examined thoroughly in the hospital in Passau. Result: If it got worse, I would have to be treated with medicines or by treating the nerve cells in the heart. **The rhythm disturbance got worse with time. My physical performance was often reduced to below 70%.**

I didn't dare leave the house any more.

In November 1996, after studying your book, I immediately began a vitamin regimen. After three weeks (9 tablets per day) the **cardiac rhythm disturbance had disappeared. It has never returned.**

After half a year, even the breathing difficulties that came with exercise were gone.

Nitrospray was no longer necessary. Now after 18 months I can, at the age of 68, again go mountain walking. I also work in my business every day.

In the meantime I have completely lost faith in conventional medicine.

As a businessman I have really no objection to people wanting to make money. But it should **not be at the cost of someone else's health** as happens now with orthodox medicine.

Yours sincerely,

H.R.

Dear Dr. Rath,

I am 78 years old and have suffered for five years from cardiac rhythm disorders and also from diabetes for a year. Attacks of dizziness, physical debility, thrombosis, and pulmonary embolisms in 1993 and 1997 were constantly with me as a result of my illness.

In July 1997 I was given a pacemaker, from which I suffered greatly. In June of this year I began a comprehensive vitamin program following the suggestion in your publications.

After only eight weeks my general condition was stable, and I was more energetic and much more active. This was not the case before taking the vitamins and supplements. I could not even do work in the kitchen.

Now I am interested in everything again! On August 24th of this year I had my blood checked. **The blood sugar level was okay!**

Another example of how well I am: in August I made a 14-day bus trip to the Tyrol. I mastered this with bravura, despite differences in altitude from 800 to 2800 m.

Despite the tremendous heat and the 10-hour bus journey: **No difficulty breathing, no swollen legs, and no problems with thrombosis!**

Yours sincerely,

Erika Walther

Dear Dr. Rath,

I am 67 years old and for around 25 to 30 years I have suffered acute heart problems. These problems manifested themselves in the form of **cardiac rhythm disturbance, angina pectoris, high blood pressure, breathing difficulties, and heart pain.** A friend said your books could help.

Through a program of vitamins and minerals, I notice the following improvements in my state of health:

I hardly ever have cardiac rhythm disturbance, have no difficulty breathing during exercise, and have a much better sense of well-being. Also my blood pressure has normalized, being now 135-140/80-85 in the mornings; previously it was 170/100.

As a result of this, I can take weaker and fewer medicines.

Furthermore, for many years I had suffered acute pain over my entire **spine**. Since taking the vitamins, **these symptoms too are as good as nonexistent.**

I feel much more capable.

Yours sincerely,

Günter Seidler

Dear Dr. Rath,

In the summer of this year I learned of the Cellular Health program. I have always been interested in natural therapy through my profession (chemist).

Since I was 19 I have suffered from disorders of the autonomic heart and circulatory system.

My husband has been suffering from cardiac rhythm disorders for over 20 years and has swallowed a great deal of medicine in that time. And in October of last year a coronary vessel in and to his left ventricle almost completely closed up. The heart attack was a foregone conclusion!

We have both been taking vitamins and minerals for two months.

Result: **My husband had an ECG yesterday. No circulatory disorder could be detected and no more "irregularities" are to be seen. Furthermore, his headaches are gone and the muscular cramp has disappeared.**

Although I take a somewhat smaller amount of the supplements, I have noticed a significant increase in performance. I feel neither tiredness nor exhaustion any longer.

It is a good thing that the results of your research have become more widely known and we can as a result experience an enormous improvement in the quality of life.

Yours sincerely,

Dagmar Schmidt

Dear Dr. Rath,

I am 76 years old and **have suffered from cardiac rhythm disturbance with racing of the heart** and other complaints for 20 years. There were often heavy palpitations also.

By chance, I came across your books and I have been taking vitamins and other supplements since October 1996 and since January 1997 I've taken a double dose.

After nine months I no longer had any disease, and my immune system is perfectly intact.

I don't go to the doctor any more as I no longer find it necessary. That says it all!

My three children and sons- and daughters-in-law take vitamins as a precaution.

Yours gratefully,

V.R.

Dear Dr. Rath,

I am 65 years old and for 12 years have been suffering the consequences of an obstruction in the right thigh and **from cardiac rhythm disturbance, which among other things recorded as 1,900 extra heartbeats during a long-term 24-hour ECG.** In addition, seven years ago I developed **angina pectoris problems and high blood pressure**, gradually **rising to 185/95.**

The problems associated with this were kept under control by regularly taking the medications "Lopirin Cor" and "Jenacard retard" prescribed by my GP.

But the rhythm disorders, more intense at night, frequently prevented me from sleeping normally and led, in conjunction with the angina pectoris problems, to tiredness during the day, loss of performance, and lack of drive.

In September of last year I heard your lecture with great interest, and read your books, and since October I have been a grateful user of vitamins and other supplements.

It has been possible meanwhile to cut the dosage of "Lopirin Cor" in half.

After taking the supplements for about two months, the nighttime cardiac rhythm disturbance in particular reduced markedly, normal sleep was again possible, and the daytime tiredness, loss in performance, and lack of drive disappeared.

Now in August, after ten months, all that is left of the **angina pectoris complaints** is a slight burning sensation under the breastbone, and I can speak of a healthy condition that I haven't known in many years.

My GP was able to confirm this success, among other things, through a significantly improved ECG in March and blood pressure reduced to 168/77.

Many thanks,

Yours sincerely,

H. Schier.

Dear Dr. Rath,

Because of your books I have been taking vitamins and other supplements now for about one year and I have noticed a great improvement in my health.

I am 43 years old and have always felt my **heart galloping from time to time, sometimes with a stabbing pain in the left side of my heart.**

Both these symptoms have now disappeared completely. I feel considerably better. My dizzy spells have also diminished.

I also suffered from problems with connective tissue and for years my **hemorrhoids** from straining at stool used to cause me great discomfort. Creams brought only temporary relief from the burning and itching. I was at my wit's end. Since June 22 of this year I have taken nutritional supplements faithfully. **After just one month, these annoying problems from hemorrhoids had disappeared,** although I still spend a lot of time sitting at my desk.

Now to the **circulation problems** in my legs. Here, too, symptoms such as stabbing pains, a dragging sensation, and unpleasant pulsating sensations, especially in the left leg, have disappeared completely. I can even feel a pleasant tingling in my feet right down to my toes, and I can tell very clearly that the blood is circulating through my **feet** as they have become **nice and warm again, just like my hands.**

Yours sincerely,

Arnold Andreas Neumann

Dear Dr. Rath,

I am 45 years old and for five years I have suffered from an **irregular heartbeat.** Every time I did **physical work, no matter how minor,** my heartbeat became completely irregular. At work I was always suffering from a **loss of energy.**

I heard you speak and read your publications and for three months now I have been taking vitamins and minerals in my diet.

Already after three weeks I noticed that these feelings of exhaustion had become a thing of the past and that I had a lot more energy.

Even after physical exertion I no longer suffer from any signs of irregular heartbeat.

I have no trouble getting a good night's sleep, and at times when I used to be very prone to sinusitis, my health is now fully unimpaired.

Thank you!

Yours sincerely,

R. M.

Dear Dr. Rath,

I am 77 years old and have been **suffering for 18 years** from problems with an **irregular heartbeat.** Upon the slightest physical exertion I experienced **severe pains in the chest.** Most of all I had problems with my circulation. I have also had a heart attack.

I saw your book on Cellular Health, read it, and the others, and since February of this year I have been on a program of vitamins and other dietary supplements.

After three weeks the pains in my heart had almost disappeared. I also noticed that I could **breathe much more freely** and that the pains in my legs had subsided. I have informed my doctor of this improvement in my health.

As far as my general health is concerned, I am very satisfied and **am able to do many things that used to be impossible, such as gardening, housework, and many other things.**

Yours sincerely,

Linda Neuber

Dear Dr. Rath,

I am 64 years old and for twelve years I have been suffering from **coronary pains** and high blood pressure, with sickness and an **irregular heartbeat.** I also used to suffer from feelings of anxiety.

Even after having my blood vessels dilated several times in the heart clinic at Bad Neustadt (1988-1992), I still didn't experience any real improvement. My feelings of nausea became more and more frequent, probably as a result of all the medication I was taking at the time—**Isoket retard, Adalat, Xanef, Godamet, and beta-blockers. These had the additional side effects of causing bleeding in the gullet and fainting attacks.**

Since March 1 of last year I have been taking vitamins and minerals convinced by the research you published.

After about three months I noticed that the times when I would suffer from an irregular heartbeat were becoming much less frequent. **After eight months had passed these disturbances in rhythm had gone completely and my blood pressure had dropped to what has now become an average of 150/90.**

Gradually I have been able to stop taking all my medication!

All my pains have vanished completely!

Yours sincerely,

E. M.

Dear Dr. Rath,

After my physical collapse in November of 1996 I was admitted to Lukas Hospital in Altenkirchen. Doctors discovered I was suffering from **acute irregularities of the heartbeat and dysfunctional blood pressure and pulse.** After I had stopped taking medication, I was discharged with the recommendation that I undergo cardiac catheterization. This was carried out in January of 1997 at the University Clinic in Bonn. I was prescribed medication in the following doses: 1x Norvasc 5mg, 1x Aspirin 100, fi Bisaprolol 5, 1x Cranoc 20, and 1x Isoket retard 20.

I was able to tolerate these medicines fairly well, but my **ability to work normally and to carry out usual tasks** was severely restricted.

In May of 1997 I read your book. As a result, I began taking vitamins in June of 1997.

Even after six months I was able to work better.

In the fall of 1997, following my doctor's recommendation, I attended a heart clinic for an examination of my heart. The results were so good that I was able to stop taking Isoket retard 20.

After a further examination by my own doctor in June of 1998, all of my body's readings were **back to normal.** Even my **blood pressure had returned to normal, 130 to 85/90 on average.**

An exercise ECG examination was carried out. The doctors found that there were no heartbeat irregularities or thickening of the heart muscle.

When I mentioned the vitamin program to the cardiologist, he said that he had heard about it and it was safe to assume that my good state of general health was a result of the Cellular Health Program. He recommended that I carry on with the supplements.

In closing, I must say that I am very pleased with the effectiveness of vitamins and that I am sure it has done me good. I feel so well that I am now able to play soccer again. I have recommended vitamins to two friends and have meanwhile noted an improvement in their health.

Yours sincerely,

Bernd Jung

Dear Dr. Rath,

I am 63 years old and have been suffering for six years from an **irregular pulse.** Once or twice every month I experienced **severe alterations in my heartbeat that would last from three to four hours.** It was the anxiety states that would sometimes make me **lose consciousness for several seconds** that caused me the most distress. On a few occasions I experienced panic attacks. In January of this year it became so bad that I had to go into the hospital.

The beta-blockers I was prescribed did me no good whatsoever, and my body did not respond to them at all well.

I read all your books and since March of this year I have been taking vitamins and minerals.

After four weeks I noticed that the irregularity in my heartbeat had gone altogether. I am now able to stand the heat and enjoy a glass of wine again from time to time.

I hope very much that many people will become interested in finding out about the Cellular Health program, since from what I see around me and read about in the papers, half the world seems to be ill.

Best regards,

Renate Braun

Dear Dr. Rath,

For exactly four weeks now I have been taking vitamins and minerals. I am 43 years old, and as a self-employed person I am under a great deal of stress.

After about two weeks my irregular pulse started to become normal again, and after three weeks all symptoms had disappeared completely.

My mother suffered a cerebral infarction recently, and I am happy to be able to give her the vitamin therapy, too. I am eager to see if—and how—her condition will change for the better. What is certain is that during her course of traditional medical treatment, my mother wasn't taking any additional vitamins.

Conventional medicine always tackles the symptoms and never the causes. Your work with Cellular Health gets to the root of the cause.

In these days of fast foods, I hope that many other people will realize just how important it is to take the right combination of vitamins.

Thank you!

Yours sincerely,

Thomas Funke

Dear Dr. Rath,

Since reading your books, I started taking vitamins and other supplements because no doctor, not even a super-specialist, has been able to diagnose the reasons for my high blood pressure that crops up from time to time. To start with, I was disappointed, since an instance of high blood pressure had subsided just before I started with the Cellular health program.

I nevertheless began supplementing my diet, and to my astonishment I have to say that **after two weeks my irregular pulse had almost completely disappeared,** a chronic condition that according to heart specialists was nonpathological.

Beforehand, my heart would skip a beat between **three and ten times a minute.** After these two weeks, it hardly skips a beat **once every minute;** in other words it is behaving very normally.

Yours sincerely,

M. L.

Dear Dr. Rath,

I am 70 years old and for ten years I have been suffering from a **rapid pulse**. One of my heart valves is calcified, and I suffer from occasional **pains in the heart**. I also suffer from shortness of breath when climbing stairs.

I have been taking beta-blockers for many years (medication to lower the blood pressure). This medication has a bad effect on me—my hair falls out, I suffer from nightmares, and I often have hallucinations and flickering in front of my eyes. My daughter read your book to me and I saw the light.

Since July of this year I have been taking vitamins and minerals, starting with light doses.

After four to five weeks I can say that my shortness of breath has become considerably better and the pains in my heart have almost gone.

Yours sincerely,

G. S.

Dear Dr. Rath,

I am a 75-year old woman and I am very glad and grateful that I have discovered the Cellular Health program, because **vitamins have given me new energy.** I seize every opportunity I can to tell others about my positive experience.

I suffered from high blood pressure, going up to more than 200, irregular pulse, weakness of the heart, and high cholesterol levels.

After I had suffered a slight **heart attack** in June of last year, I had an operation on the left-side carotid artery. In November, doctors discovered **that my right carotid artery was also almost closed up and would soon have to be operated on.**

However, after I had been taking vitamins for four months, **my surgeon carried out an ultrasonic examination and found that my arteries are now completely clear.**

My blood pressure is back to normal, my irregular pulse is back to normal, and I feel just like I used to years ago.

I used to have to take nine traditional medicine tablets per day; nowadays I take just four.

Before I started taking the vitamins, I tried talking about your program with my **doctor,** but she just wouldn't hear of it. But after she had **received the positive report written by my surgeon she was quite amazed** and has started reading your book "Why Animals Don't Get Heart Attacks" and listening to your Chemnitz cassette with great interest.

I can only repeat that I have derived enormous benefit from the vitamins and would like to thank you once again for this result.

When I was really feeling at my lowest, I took a higher dose for a few days and felt so much better.

Many thanks to you for your research work!

Yours sincerely,

F. M.

Dear Dr. Rath,

I am 46 years old. Four years ago I had a kidney transplant and in April of 1996, I had a heart attack. Because of your research I have been on vitamin therapy for one year now, two.

After just four weeks I was starting to feel better, and the massive problems I had with my irregular heartbeat disappeared almost immediately.

Yours sincerely,

M. Müller

7

Diabetes
and Diabetic Circulatory
Problems

Cellular Health
for Natural Prevention
and Health Maintenance

The Facts About Adult Diabetes

Worldwide over one hundred million people are suffering from diabetes. Diabetic disorders have a genetic background and are divided into two types: juvenile and adult onset diabetes. Juvenile diabetes is generally caused by an inborn defect that leads to insufficient insulin in the body and requires regular insulin injections to control blood sugar levels. The majority of diabetic patients, however, develop this disease as adults. Adult forms of diabetes also have a genetic background. The causes, however, that trigger the outbreak of the disease in these patients at any stage of their adult lives, have been unknown. It is, therefore, not surprising thatdiabetes is yet another disease that is still expanding on a worldwide scale.

Conventional medicine is confined to treating the symptoms of adult diabetes by lowering elevated blood sugar levels. However, cardiovascular diseases and other diabetic complications occur even in those patients with controlled blood sugar levels. Thus, lowering of blood sugar levels is a necessary but an insufficient and incomplete treatment of diabetic disorders.

Modern Cellular Health now provides a breakthrough in our understanding of the causes, the prevention, and the adjunct therapy of adult diabetes. Adult onset diabetes is frequently caused or aggravated by a deficiency of certain vitamins and other essential nutrients in millions of cells in the pancreas, the liver, and the blood vessel walls.This deficiency of nutrients can trigger a diabetic metabolism and the onset of adult diabetes in people with a genetic predisposition to diabetic disorders. Vice versa, optimum intake of vitamins and other nutrients can help prevent the onset of adult diabetes and correct, at least in part, existing diabetes and its complications.

Diabetes-Related Cardiovascular Problems and Circulatory Disorders

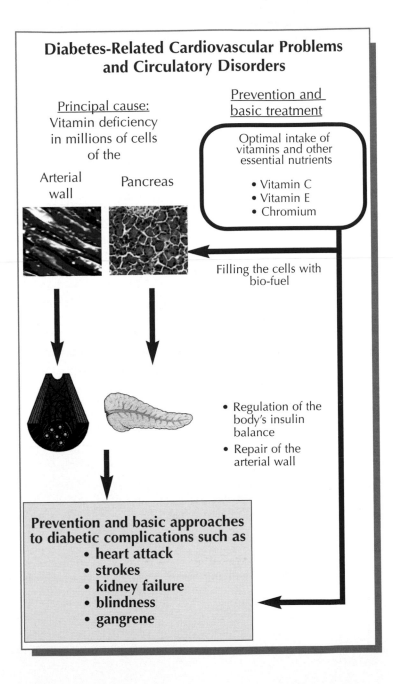

Principal cause:
Vitamin deficiency in millions of cells of the

Prevention and basic treatment

Arterial wall

Pancreas

Optimal intake of vitamins and other essential nutrients

- Vitamin C
- Vitamin E
- Chromium

Filling the cells with bio-fuel

- Regulation of the body's insulin balance
- Repair of the arterial wall

Prevention and basic approaches to diabetic complications such as
- **heart attack**
- **strokes**
- **kidney failure**
- **blindness**
- **gangrene**

Dear Dr. Rath,

I am 42 years of age and have had **diabetes for two years now**. The effects are tiredness, thirst, and glucose in the urine. Most of all I have suffered from **a lack of vitality.**

I needed help. Then I found your books. Since May of this year I have been taking vitamins and minerals. **After just two weeks my blood sugar level was** so **normal** that I feel completely well without taking Manninil.

It is the improvement in my general health that has pleased me most of all.

My **doctor confirmed this improvement** when he measured a constant normalization of my blood sugar level.

Yours sincerely,

R. W.

Dear Dr. Rath,

I am 75 years old and have been a diabetic for many years. About one year ago my **blood sugar level** went up enormously. It **fluctuated between 15 and 17 mmol/l (270 - 305 mg/dl)**. The doctor who was treating me wanted me to change over to insulin injections, but I did not want that.

With the knowledge from your books I began taking the food supplements, extra vitamins and minerals. It was still possible for me to switch over to insulin injections at any time if there was no improvement in my blood sugar levels.

However, I hardly dared believe that **after just a short time** of regularly taking the supplements, **my blood sugar level had dropped. It now fluctuates between 6.5 and 9.5 mmol/l (117 to 171)**. But if that weren't enough, my **whole well-being** has improved enormously. You can imagine how happy I am about this, since **it means I don't have to have injections.**

I am extremely happy with my current general health. I would be very pleased if many other people suffering from diabetes were able to improve their health problems with a vitamin program, or even be completely cured.

Yours sincerely,

H. S.

Dear Dr. Rath,

I am 69 years old and have been suffering from **high blood pressure for 20 years. For three years I have also been suffering from diabetes.** During this time I have suffered from symptoms that have increased as time has gone on, such as general tiredness and lack of interest, and stiff joints. Later on I suffered from **cold and numb toes.**

My friend told me about your work. Since June 25th of this year I began a program to supplement my diet with vitamins and minerals.

After only three weeks the feeling came back in my toes and my feet, and they felt warm again.

I have also become more supple again, and I can do jobs I'm not used to doing without any difficulty or pain.

I am fit again; **it's been a long while since I felt as well as I do now!**

Yours sincerely,

Klaus Schumacher

Dear Dr. Rath,

I am 60 years old and have suffered from **diabetes for six years.** My symptoms have been **difficulties in seeing properly, scurfy patches on my skin, bleeding gums, tiredness and thirst.** It was feeling tired during the day that was the most unpleasant for me.

Your books gave me hope that i could become healthy and since May of last year I have been taking vitamins and minerals.

After three weeks I regained my full sight, and my other symptoms have nearly all disappeared.

I hope a lot of people will get to hear about the benefits of vitamins. I will do my bit to make that happen.

Yours sincerely,

Jürgen Schäfer

Dear Dr. Rath,

I am 75 years old. As well as having **diabetes**, a year ago I suffered a stroke. But the worst problem for me was **poor circulation in my legs.**

For four weeks now I have been taking vitamins and other nutritional supplements described in your book.

After this period of time I can say that t**he circulation in my legs has improved and that my blood sugar levels have gone down to 100-113 mg/dl.**

When he saw this improvement in my health, my **doctor was at a loss for words,** especially as he had already been considering the possibility of **amputating my legs.**

I can do light housework again, such as ironing and cooking.

I owe this to my daughter, Ute Heinz, and my friends; they are the ones who introduced me to Cellular Health and made me enjoy life again.

Yours sincerely,

Edeltraud Heinz

Dear Dr. Rath,

Studying your book led me to thoroughly re-think my health situation. I have always been interested in medical problems, but now I have been thinking about these things in a new intensity and depth—as far as a technical person is able to understand medicine.

I am 67 years old and suffer from hereditary diabetes mellitus, heart problems, and weak arteries. I have doctors' certificates attesting to the following illnesses:

- **Diabetes mellitus with complications** (1970 diabetes manifest, discovered by my dentist as a result of severe bleeding of the gums and periodontitis, with **four operations on my gums—it was the beginnings of scurvy!)**

- Cerebro-vascular deficiency (inadequate circulation of blood in the brain)

- Reduced heart output with coronary cardiopathy and **high blood pressure** (1976-1990 increased levels of up to 180/100; 1990/91 **heart attacks,** 1994 treatment by a heart specialist with 75 mg Atenolol, 40 mg Mifedipin, 10 mg ACE inhibitors, 100 mg AS5 per day, and in emergencies Nitro-Spray; 1996 extreme loss of vitality)

- Constantly **swollen ankles and lower legs,** fluid in both my shins; in 1997 my blood pressure fell to 90/58 with a pulse of 49

- **Peripheral circulatory disorders** (in the limbs)

- Although I am very careful about what I eat (I am almost a vegetarian), have lost nine lbs. and weigh just one lbs. more than my ideal weight, I have very high **cholesterol levels, from 190 to 250 mg/dl.**

In addition to these problems, I also suffered from **neuropathic dysfunction (damage to the nerves) in my feet, with severe numbness**—I no longer had any feeling when pricked with a pin—loss of balance, and what is sometimes called "window-shopping legs," with frequent cramps and pains in my legs and feet. Occasionally I suffered from autonomous nervous disorders.

After I had been taking vitamins since February of this year, and reading your book, I learned in May about the health network and am currently supplementing my diet with further nutrients.

I have been taking the vitamins therapy for six months now and can report the following:

- In cooperation with my doctor I have been able to stop taking all the calcium antagonists, the beta-blockers, ACE inhibitors, and AS 5, as well as the diuretics. I am still taking 16 mg of a Ansiotensin II receptor blockers and 100 mg of Pentoxifyllin.

- **The pains and cramps in my legs have disappeared and the first signs of feeling are starting to come back in my feet,** tests with a microfilament give positive results in four places. I have sensation on the soles of my feet again when I am tickled there, but I still have some pain.

- **The autonomous neuropathies have receded.** I am able to walk around town again without first having to plan toilet stops.

- My physical strength has increased considerably. **In January I needed to stop six to eight times in order to walk up a 200 m path with a 13% slope; now I can complete the distance briskly without having to stop at all.** It used to take me 65 minutes in January to walk a certain distance on the flat; now I can complete the distance in 45 minutes.

- As for the diabetes treatment, I had the option to stop taking either 5 mg of **Glibenclamid or 10 units of prolonged action insulin.** I decided to stop taking the pill.

- All the measures I was taking to combat my high cholesterol level have allowed me to stop the **cholesterol depressants.** My doctor was pleased with this development, too.

- The **pulse in my feet** has been clearly evident again for about six weeks now; this is an enormous step forward for me.

I am firmly resolved to continue this course of treatment. I shall put the motto "Patience is the key to joy" up on the wall. I shall report back to you again in a few months' time.

With my sincerest thanks and best wishes,

Yours,

Dr. K. G. W.

Dear Dr. Rath,

Since May of this year I have been taking vitamins and minerals described in your publications and have met with great success.

In 1997 I suffered a slight stroke and have as a result had to undergo an operation to the carotid artery.

I have been registered as a **category II diabetic since 1984.**

In the past few months, the HBA 1 value (the laboratory test for the mean **blood sugar level** taken over the last 2-3 weeks) has gone down considerably from 9.6 to 6.2.

The circulation in my legs and feet has also improved visibly. On the whole, I am able to walk much better.

Kind regards,

W. B.

Dear Dr. Rath,

I am 56 years old and have suffered from diabetes for ten years. My blood sugar count was measured at **between 9.0 and 14.0 mmol/l (160 to 250 mg/dl).**

Vitamins helped my son. He gave me your books. Since January of this year I have been taking vitamins and other supplements. My blood sugar count is now between **4.0 and 8.0 mmol/l (70 to 140 mg/dl).**

With my doctor's approval, I have been able to reduce the medicines I was taking to treat the diabetes.

Yours sincerely,

Egon Stölzel

Dear Dr. Rath,

For two weeks now I have been taking vitamins and minerals described in your book.

I no longer suffer from **cramps in my feet**, the continuous twitching has stopped, and beforehand I was unable to keep my right foot still because of the continuous pain day and night.

When I began the vitamin therapy, the sugar count went up slightly; it then went down considerably.

Yours sincerely,

F. K.

Dear Dr. Rath,

I am 58 years of age and have suffered for about five years from the **late symptoms of diabetes: loss of sight, circulatory disorders with diabetic gangrene in the feet** (they told me they might have to consider amputation), **high blood pressure**, serious heart problems, and very poor renal values.

After I had heard a report on Bavarian radio, I immediately went out and bought your book.

For about two years now I have been supplementing my diet with vitamins and minerals. After about twelve months I noticed the following improvement in my general state of health:

- **Constant blood pressure**,

- **Improved renal values (as a result, I was able to avoid having to undergo dialysis treatment just in the nick of time)**,

- **Almost completely healed feet, with the prevention of what looked like unavoidable amputation of my legs.**

My positive experiences mean that I am able to recommend vitamins to other people without the slightest reservation.

Yours sincerely,

Walter Habermann

Dear Dr. Rath,

I have been a diabetic for more than 40 years now. I read about Cellular Health and began treatment with a high dosage of vitamins and other supplements, I am able to see the first positive results.

I feel fit and well and note **an improvement in my polyneuropathy** (polyneuropathy is damage to the nerves, typical for diabetics; it can lead to a lack of feeling and numbness, especially in the legs).

I was in danger of losing a toe on my right foot—and yesterday my doctor found that the condition had improved.

I am pleased to be able to tell you that vitamin therapy has enabled me to combat the diabetes and improve my general state of health.

Thank you very much.

Yours sincerely,

E. B.

Dear Dr. Rath,

I would like to start off by thanking you from the bottom of my heart for your work.

I am 76 years old and have suffered from **diabetes** since 1977. My GP has treated me with pills over many years. In the course of the years, my feet and **legs and lower legs turned nearly dark blue.**

In 1991 I was **paralyzed down the left side of my face.** My left eye, left nostril, and the left part of my lower lip were most affected by the **damage caused to my nerves.**

I have been taking vitamins since March of this year.

My condition improved after just eight weeks. At the present moment in time I can report the following:

1. **It is now impossible to detect the damage to my left eye.** My eyelid does not droop anymore, and the feeling of having a completely dry eye has all but gone.

2. The symptoms of the damage caused to my lower lip were a continuous feeling of **dryness and numbness.** Both these symptoms have **disappeared completely.**

3. The left part of my **nose** was always dry and I had no feeling in it. Today, everything is back to **normal again.**

4. I had serious problems with the **circulation in my lower legs and feet.** I always suffered from cold feet. Dark patches had started to form on the insides of my ankles because my feet were not getting enough blood.

Today, **my feet are warm again and my circulation is normal.** The dark patches on my left foot have become lighter; on my right foot the patches have become a lot lighter.

5. My **daily blood sugar count** (measured with rods and blood) **is almost normal again.**

I can hardly tell you how grateful I am. Thanks to the supplements, I am able to enjoy a good quality of life again. I am greatly encouraged.

The only thing I really regret is that I did not find out about the benefits of vitamins until now, now that I am in old age. I am quite convinced that my problems could have been avoided if I had known about vitamins earlier.

I can warmly recommend anyone who is suffering from diabetes to begin taking supplements as soon as possible. I have told all my friends, neighbors, and all the doctors and pharmacists I know about your research. I have also passed on the books and other material I have for other people to read.

My hope for millions of other people is that they hear about vitamin therapy as soon as possible so that illnesses can be prevented and suffering reduced.

I wish you lots of energy for your continued work. I hope that one day you will have the success you deserve with your admirable work.

Again, thank you very much.

Yours sincerely,

W. G.

1

Dear Dr. Rath,

I have been a category II diabetic for 16 years now and have been injecting myself with insulin for 14 years. Before I started a vitamin program, I was an ill-adjustable diabetic. Your books changed the way I looked at health.

My blood sugar count was very high, fluctuating between good and bad. At the time, my long-term HbA 1c value was 8.4.

In March of this year I began taking vitamin and mineral supplements in my diet.

Not only did my metabolic process start to stabilize, but I even managed to achieve **optimal values.** There is no doubt about this whatsoever; we only need to refer to my **blood sugar count!** My current HbA 1c long-term value is 6.6.

- 2 -

I have also been able to reduce my intake of insulin by about one third. In the course of time, one of the added benefits of this will be the saving in cost to my health insurance company.

Although I can still be classed as an intensive user of insulin, taking the new "Humalog" drug, I maintain that the vitamin therapy has contributed to the improvement in my blood sugar levels and to the overall improvement in my general state of health.

I shall continue taking the nutritional supplements with the insulin. On the strength of my positive experiences I can recommend it to all diabetics who might be interested.

Yours sincerely,

Günter Behm

Dear Dr. Rath,

Diabetes runs in my family, both sides, and my mother suffers badly from it. She takes insulin and has had problems with the circulation in her feet. The doctors wanted to cut off her toes. Things were getting bad. I didn't want my mom to be without toes.

Then I was diagnosed with diabetes. In my youth I had been somewhat of an athlete and remembered that the body responds to good nutrition. Your books helped me, and I began a program that supplemented my diet with vitamins and minerals.

Within six weeks I felt the changes and had my doctor run some further tests. He confirmed that the supplements had improved my health. I took your research and the results of my tests to my mother and they helped convince her to start vitamin therapy.

Today I am delighted to say that both me and mother are feeling wonderful. Her toes are toasty warm now and she wears sandals in the good weather. She likes to show off her painted toenails.

Thanks to you and for your research into the benefits of vitamins.

Yours in Good Health,

L.F

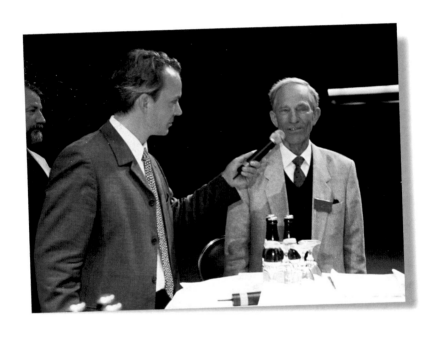

Patients lined up to tell of their freedom from pharmaceutical drugs.

8

Other Diseases

- **Varicose Veins**
- **Asthma**
- **Skin Disorders**
- **Eye Diseases**
- **Headaches**

**Cellular Health
Addresses
Other Common Illnesses**

VARICOSE VEINS

Dear Dr. Rath,

I am 42 years old and have been suffering from **varicose veins for six years.** I have been continuously plagued by severe pain in my legs and **cramps in my calf muscles** at night.

I saw your literature and four months ago I began taking vitamins and minerals. **After just eight weeks the nighttime attacks of cramps had become a thing of the past** and I was even able to walk and stand for longer periods of time without experiencing any pain.

I am immensely impressed by the vitamin therapy and have already recommended it to many others.

Yours sincerely,

Gabriele Winkler

Dear Dr. Rath,

Since learning about Cellular Health, I decided to take charge of my life, and for about five weeks now I have been supplementing my diet with vitamins and minerals and other beneficial nutrients.

The vitamin therapy has improved my digestion; cholesterol greatly reduced to normal levels.

My circulation has improved; left foot lets me sleep at night without bothering me; before, I was always in pain from my varicose veins. Now, my varicose **veins are receding,** and I am free of pain.

My nerves are better, and my general health has improved considerably.

Because of these fantastic results, I can warmly recommend vitamin therapy to everyone; in fact, this is something that I do very actively.

Yours sincerely,

B. K.

Dear Dr. Rath,

I read your books and I have been taking vitamins and minerals for eight weeks now.

I have suffered for several years from internal **varicose veins** and have already undergone an operation for them (about 10 years ago). However, varicose veins occurred again in the same spot. At times they were so sensitive that even a blanket over my feet caused me severe pain.

Just three days after beginning the vitamin regimem, I noticed a considerable improvement in sensitivity, and after one week I was free of pain.

Even during my first period after I had begun the supplements, I no longer suffered from **menstrual pains** (before I used to have a dragging sensation in my lower abdomen and backache).

Yours sincerely,

B. K.

Dear Dr. Rath,

I am 37 years old and have suffered from **swollen legs** for four years. After I had had an inflamed wound, my leg was red with scars and swollen because of an **accumulation of fluid.** Standing and walking caused me the most pain.

Your research looked valid and in March of this year I began taking vitamins and minerals; after two months I began to notice an improvement in my health.

The swelling in my legs has **almost completely disappeared** and the scars and patches have become smaller, too.

Even my varicose veins are receding. I hope I will be able to tell many more people about the effects of the vitamin therapy.

Yours sincerely,

B. G.

ASTHMA

Dear Dr. Rath,

I am 62 years old and have been suffering from **bronchial asthma** for 25 years, together with colds (neglected flu). Most of all I have been suffering from **asthma attacks** and attendant **shortness of breath.**

Since April of this year I have been taking vitamins and mineral supplements I learned about from your book.

After eleven weeks I no longer had to use my inhaler, which before had been my constant companion. I was able to breathe freely once again.

This is the best thing that could possibly happen to me!

Yours sincerely,

Marianne Stein

Dear Dr. Rath,

I was born in 1924 and until I reached the age of 60 I was bothered by few health problems. Then I became very ill, and the doctors diagnosed life-threatening **anemia** and **asthma**. Despite many examinations, the cause for my anemia could not be determined. For almost ten years I had to receive one or two blood transfusions a year. Although the hemoglobin value improved during the last three years, it still went up and down a lot.

I often suffered tremendous **shortness of breath as a result of the asthma.**

My friend told me of your work and the great strides you made in health. Since the beginning of the year I have been taking dietary supplements.

Over the last few weeks I have noticed a **clear improvement in my health** and I am very pleased that my blood readings taken in April and on August 22nd of this year show very good, stable values.

My asthma has improved too.

Best regards,

Gudrun Heumann

Dear Dr. Rath,

I am 56 years old and have suffered from **bronchial asthma** for almost ten years. The illness began with a flu-type infection with severe bronchitis, for which my GP prescribed "Allergospasmin" inhaler (a medicine in spray form designed to relieve the spasms of the small air cells in the lungs).

Since that time, I was **unable to leave the house,** sometimes not even the room, **without having this medicine with me.** On good days, I needed to inhale it "only" every three to seven hours. Whenever I had a flu-type infection, I often needed to use it every one to one-and-a-half hours, day and night. **I was often on the verge of suffocating.**

I have tried all sorts of treatments, both alternative natural methods and antibiotics, cortisone, and anti-allergic agents. Nothing was really able to help. Since I could almost set my watch by the length of time between the shortness of breath attacks, I had long been convinced that I had developed a medication dependency.

I wanted natural treatments and found your publications. For three months (i.e., since June 2nd of this year) I have been on a vitamin regimen.

2

After four weeks, I started to lengthen the time between my aerosol inhalations. It was a real withdrawal for me and more or less a torture, but it got better and better.

One whole week passed before the last time I had to inhale, and that's now two months ago. Occasionally I would still suffer some shortness of breath, but I stuck it out, and from day to day these attacks became less bothersome and more infrequent. My suspicion that I had had for years, that a weak heart and irregularity of the heartbeat were the basic causes of my asthma, was confirmed; these had receded into the background because of the relaxing effect of the asthma preparations.

Since January I have added more supplements and, and my **recovery is progressing by leaps and bounds.**

I still can't believe that shortness of breath and medicine dependency are things of the past.

This is a new life for me! Thank you, Dr. Rath!

Yours sincerely,

Doris Hildebrandt

Dear Dr. Rath,

For many years I suffered from recurrent infections. I often had bronchitis twice a year. About three years ago this took the form of **spastic bronchitis.**

Since the beginning of the year I have been taking additional vitamins and minerals in my diet. This very quickly led to a solid overall improvement in my general health. **My susceptibility to infections has practically disappeared,** and I am able to cope much better with stress.

Since listening to your cassette "Basics of Cellular Health," I have also been furthering my nutritional intake.

There has since been a noticeable change in my lungs. Everything has become much **clearer, and I am able to draw really deep breaths.**

Thank you very much once again for all that you have done!

With best regards,

Gerda Tecklenburg

Dear Dr. Rath,

I have been suffering from **asthma** for many years, moreso since 1981. In 1996 I was admitted to the hospital three times with a suspected heart attack. Fortunately, this was never confirmed! The pains always began on the left side under the last rib, accompanied by a shortness of breath. Through dedicated care and the use of the latest technology together with all types of medication, I was able to leave the hospital on each occasion. I was given **oxygen equipment,** and this helped me to accomplish my everyday household chores.

I am also suffering from a build up of fluid in my legs. At Dresden Heart Clinic my daily intake of fluid was set at 1.5 litres. But the water still remained in my legs.

It was only on the recommendation of a non-medical practitioner who was treating me, and your books, that I started vitamin therapy; **the swelling in my legs has gone down enormously;** when the weather is cooler the swelling often disappears altogether.

At the same time my general health has improved. I have been able to manage for **weeks now without inhalers**. A trip into the hills climbing up 100 metres is no problem for me at all, and at home I am no longer afraid to climb up two floors to go into the loft.

This is a marvellous success after only six months!

Yours sincerely,

J. N.

SKIN / PSORIASIS / ALLERGIES

Dear Dr. Rath,

I have been a member of your network since January of this year. For 22 years I have suffered from **psoriasis** and have been under the treatment of dermatologists.

In February I heard about your lectures. At that time I had patches of psoriasis the **size of my palm**, on both elbows, on both knees, and on my head. I sought the help of a nutritional advisor in your network. She recommended I take a zinc preparation together with vitamins and minerals. I followed her advice and started taking the zinc preparation, one capsule mornings and evenings. Shortly afterwards I began taking the Cellular Health vitamins.

It is now October, and with the exception of a tiny spot on my scalp, I have been free of this bothersome complaint for about two weeks now. **My arms and legs are smooth again, as if they never had anything wrong with them.** I would therefore like to take this opportunity to thank you, Dr. Rath, and your advisor for your help. Since I know there are many people suffering from this disease, I would like for them, too, to learn about your wonderful method. I am therefore quite happy for you to publish my letter.

Yours sincerely,

Wolfgang Horn

Dear Dr. Rath,

I am 51 years of age. I have suffered for 30 years from a **pollen allergy** that begins every year in April and goes away again sometime in July. Frequent **flu-type infections** and difficulty in breathing are always a continuous torture for me during this time. I also used to suffer from bad backache.

Since December of last year I have been taking vitamins and minerals described in your book. After five months I have noticed the following improvements in my general health:

I no longer have any **infections** and **my allergy was nowhere near as bad as in previous years.** I am also very pleased that my backache has been reduced to a minimum.

And there's something else, too. Since my hysterectomy at the age of 38, I've had to take **hormone preparations**. When I began the vitamin therapy, I was able to **stop taking this medication.**

I feel very well!

Yours sincerely,

Helga Irmler

Dear Dr. Rath,

For three years my husband, aged 73, suffered from an allergy in **the neck, shoulder, and face region.** He also suffered from circulatory problems in his right leg. No doctor was really able to bring him any relief.

We happened upon your books and in July 10th of this year my husband started taking nutritional supplements, mainly vitamins and minerals. After just one week the itching disappeared and his nerves calmed down. Two weeks later, three quarters of his allergy had vanished. After a total of just four weeks, all that my husband had was a lymph swelling on his neck.

After four weeks he added more supplements.

The itching has gone, the allergy has gone and the circulatory problems have almost disappeared, too. My husband is his happy, jolly self again, just like he used to be before his illness.

I also had problems with high blood pressure and slight arteriosclerosis (I am 60 years of age). **My blood pressure was 200/100.** I also started taking the supplements, just like my husband, and in the same dose.

After fourteen days, my blood pressure had become normal. I feel healthy and strengthened. Through taking the vitamins and minerals, my knee and fingers have become more supple and pain free.

Thank you very much indeed. We tell everyone we meet everywhere about the Cellular Health program.

I have been a nurse for 35 years and have never before seen such results, only the misery that results from conventional medicine!

Thank you very much once again.

Yours sincerely,

Anna-Sibylla Saatz

ARTHROSIS / OSTEOPOROSIS

Dear Dr. Rath,

My mother, Mrs. Maria Kohlmann, has experienced great success with vitamin supplements. She is 75 years of age and suffers from **rheumatism.** She has pain mostly in her arms. When she tries lifting her arms it causes her great pain.

For one year she took a **cortisone preparation** prescribed by the doctor. Sometimes the medication would help to ease the pain, but she was never really free of pain.

With the help of your books, I was able to persuade her to try vitamin therapy. After about two months she reduced the amount of cortisone she was still taking because the pain had subsided considerably.

One month later she was beaming with joy as she told me how she could move **her arms again like normal, and that the pain had disappeared completely.**

She has now stopped taking cortisone completely.

Yours sincerely,

Maria Kohlmann and Rosemarie Brandl

Dear Dr. Rath,

These are the complaints I had before I read your fine books and started taking vitamins and minerals:

1. **Severe hair loss for weeks on end;** nothing that I did could stop it.

2. **Arthritis and back pain for many years** following an operation for a slipped disc. Because of this I had to use **two crutches wherever I went** at all times. Standing caused me tremendous pain and I was unable to do any housework.

3. As a result of thrombosis and cardiac insufficiency **my feet were swollen** in the evenings, despite wearing support stockings.

After I started taking the vitamin supplements, I noticed the following improvements in my general health:

1. After three days **my hair loss disappeared altogether.**

2. I am now able to work around the house **without crutches.** I am able to cook again and use both hands to carry things with. I am also able to do light housework.

3. **My legs are slim** and my shoes fit me better.

Thank you very much,

Sincerely yours,

L. D.

Dear Dr. Rath,

I am 55 years old and have suffered for 14 years from **osteoporosis**. Since I had a radical hysterectomy 14 years ago I have suffered from unbearable **backache and pain in my bones.** My posture has changed and I have become smaller.

After I had had broken bones on several occasions (comminuted fractures), the doctors diagnosed osteoporosis. I was continuously afraid of breaking bones again.

Your research and a friend convinced me to try supplements and since April of this year I have been taking vitamins and minerals .

After four months my health had improved and I was free of all pain. The fact that I am almost able to walk upright again is an enormous change. This improvement in my health has been confirmed by **new X-rays; they show that the osteoporosis has disappeared.**

I will do my bit to spread the word about your vital information on vitamin research, so that other people can be helped.

Yours sincerely,

Christine Ralle

Dear Dr. Rath,

I am 55 years old and for 10 years I have been suffering from **arthritis of the fingers.** This complaint causes a gradual **stiffening of the hands.** The recurring inflammation has given me an awful amount of pain.

I read your excellent books and in 1996 I began taking vitamins and minerals.

After 18 months I can safely say: **The pains have subsided, and above all, the times when my finger joints become inflamed** are far less frequent. My doctor has also recommended I continue taking the vitamins.

Yours sincerely,

H. J.

Dear Dr. Rath,

I am 58 years of age and have been suffering from osteoporosis for eight years. My symptoms were severe backache and pain in the joints, like a bad case of flu. I also suffered from pain in the lower abdomen.

In searching for a natural treatment, I came across your books and for six weeks I have been taking vitamins and mineral and other supplements. After three weeks my backache had reduced considerably, and the bleeding between periods stopped.

I have also been taking estrogen for 16 years (prescribed by various gynecologists). My doctor has agreed for me to stop taking this, and I feel very well with the vitamin program.

Yours sincerely,

B. W.

Dear Dr. Rath,

I am 48 years old and have had to take **estrogen** for the last two years following a **radical hysterectomy** in 1996. Hot flashes and **the start of osteoporosis in the neck region** (quite clearly visible in X-rays) were a real burden for me.

A friend who had your books lent them to me. In January of this year I began taking vitamins and minerals.

After about two months, the annoying **hot flashes had stopped** and the **pain around my neck vertebrae** had subsided considerably. I also notice that I have much more energy.

In February I was able to stop taking the **estrogen** and have been able to achieve far better results with vitamin therapy than with the hormone replacement therapy.

Yours sincerely,

Petra Bollmohr

EYE DISEASES

Dear Dr. Rath,

About one year ago I recommended that my aunt (65) in Nuremberg try some vitamins. She was sceptical and refused to consider it, having heard negative reports about it. She said she was already eating a lot of fruit and took vitamin tablets from to time.

I told her that that was not enough, and with the powerful research in your books I was finally able to convince her to try a proper regime and give her body a chance.

After about one month she phoned me to say her galloping heartbeat had completely gone. She was on cloud nine.

She also told me of the general improvement in her state of health. She had more energy and did not get so easily out of breath when jogging, like she used to do.

Before she started with the course of vitamins, her optician had diagnosed a **considerable worsening of her eye condition**. He asked her to go back for another eye examination six months later.

After a half a year on the vitamin program she went back to have her eyes tested. The doctor was amazed and said her **eyes had improved considerably.** She asked him: Doctor, how is that possible? He was lost for an answer.

Six months later she had her eyes tested again. The doctor confirmed that the **internal pressure in the eye had become normal,** and her sight had improved, too.

She revealed her secret of vitamin therapy and said she was absolutely delighted.

Today, she is a staunch defender of vitamins and your work. She feels fit and well and would never want to be without the tablets again.

Yours sincerely,

Arnold H. Neumann

HEADACHE / MIGRAINE

Dear Dr. Rath,

I am 47 years old and have suffered for 22 years from migraine. Resulting from a paralysis of the facial nerve on the right side of my face, I have suffered from **severe headaches just above my right eye** since 1977. I have also suffered many times from trigeminus neuralgia. I have sought the help from many doctors, but a lasting improvement has not been possible, merely a temporary reduction in the pain.

Nothing helped until I saw your books and since March of this year I have been taking vitamins and minerals.

After about two weeks I was experiencing periods when I was completely free of pain. The slight pains I was now having were quite bearable in comparison with what I had been used to earlier. My quality of life has improved considerably. I am able to perform tasks and do not get exhausted so quickly as before.

After all those years there were times when I just felt like giving up. But all that has changed now!

Yours sincerely,

S. S.

Dear Dr. Rath,

I am 24 years of age and have been suffering from headaches for six years. **Severe headache** would develop every time after I had indulged in heavy physical exercise and after long periods of work.

Since June of this year I have been taking vitamins, minerals and other nutrient supplements, the ones you write of in your books.

After eight weeks I noticed that **my headaches had become very rare.** What is especially noticeable was that when I do get headaches, they are very slight indeed.

Taking the supplements has vastly improved my quality of life. I am able to do a lot more! Thank you, Dr. Rath. I hope you will be able to help many people just like you have been able to help me.

Yours sincerely,

A. G.

Dear Dr. Rath,

I am 77 years of age and for many years I have suffered from **circulatory disorders** accompanied by **headaches and dizzy spells** that often prevent me from walking just a few steps.

My son's wife gave me your literature and for four months now I have been regularly taking vitamins and minerals.

For the last two months my blood pressure has gone down from 180/110 to 145/80. In addition, the **dizzy spells** have disappeared completely and the headaches have also **drastically subsided.**

It was my son who drew my attention to the Cellular Health program, and I am so glad he did.

I would also like to recommend vitamins to other people.

Yours sincerely,

Gerda Hunger

Dear Dr. Rath,

My wife, aged 38, has suffered from **bad migraines since she was a child.** The doctors simply did not know what to do, were unable to do anything more for her, and even wanted to admit her for psychiatric treatment. Fortunately, her mother was able to prevent that from happening.

Finally, my wife had to take **strong morphine-based painkillers**, and always had a supply of them in the fridge so she could be injected on short notice any time night or day. The side effects meant that she was very restricted in her job (she is in nursing).

Acute circulatory problems and the related migraine attacks meant that she was often confined to **bed for days at a time.** All the medication she was taking managed to stop the attacks, but nothing that she tried brought her any fundamental help.

That is why I did not have any faith when she began supplementing her diet with vitamins and minerals at the beginning of June this year; I just thought it would be another useless and expensive attempt at combating the illness. As a nurse, she understood your research better than I.

After just three months I was shown to be quite wrong. As early as the beginning of August she was feeling much better. Today, my wife is able to do without **some of her strong medication, and she has had no more migraine attacks**. Thank you very much!

Yours sincerely,

Mathias Dörfer

Dear Dr. Rath,

I am 35 years old and have been suffering from **bad headaches** for ten years. I would particularly suffer from them in stress situations and if I was not getting enough sleep. The pains were really awful.

My friend told me about you and your work and in March this year I began taking minerals and vitamins.

Eight weeks later my headaches had left me completely. After a long day at work I am no longer as tense as I used to be.

I am so grateful that I found out about vitamin therapy, that I am able to use it, and that it has done me good.

Yours sincerely,

Kerstin Mende

You can find further up-to-date information about vitamin research and Cellular Health in Dr. Rath's best sellers from the Cellular Health series **The Heart, Cancer, and Ten Years that Changed Medicine Forever** as well as on the Internet.

Our Internet address **www.drrath.com** has become one of the world's most frequently consulted sources of information on natural health.

Every day thousands of people all over the world visit the site in their quest for essential information—information they can find nowhere else.

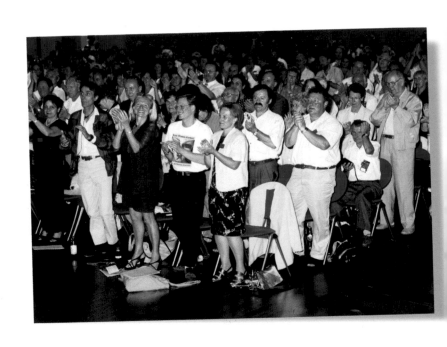